Shoulder Pain

The Therapy for Shoulder and Neck Pain

(The Solution & Prevention of Shoulder Pain in Just 5 Minutes)

Eugene Franklin

Published By **Jackson Denver**

Eugene Franklin

Shoulder Pain: The Therapy for Shoulder and Neck Pain (The Solution & Prevention of Shoulder Pain in Just 5 Minutes)

ISBN   978-1-998769-31-5

Legal & Disclaimer

The information contained in this ebook is not designed to replace or take the place of any form of medicine or professional medical advice. The information in this ebook has been provided for educational & entertainment purposes only.

The information contained in this book has been compiled from sources deemed reliable, and it is accurate to the best of the Author's knowledge; however, the Author cannot guarantee its accuracy and validity and cannot be held liable for any errors or omissions. Changes are periodically made to this book. You must consult your doctor or get professional medical advice before using any of the suggested remedies, techniques, or information in this book.

Upon using the information contained in this book, you agree to hold harmless the Author from and against any damages, costs, and expenses, including any legal fees potentially resulting from the application of any of the information provided by this guide. This disclaimer applies to any damages or injury caused by the use and application, whether directly or indirectly, of any advice or information presented, whether for breach of contract, tort, negligence, personal injury, criminal intent, or under any other cause of action.

You agree to accept all risks of using the information presented inside this book. You need to consult a professional medical practitioner in order to ensure you are both able and healthy enough to participate in this program.

Table Of Contents

Chapter 1: The Muscle And Neck Stretches

To Help Muscle The Pain

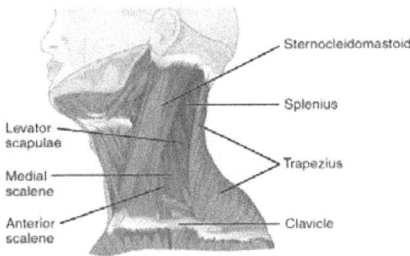

The muscles in your neck are numerous which include the levator scapulae muscle as well as erector spinae, sternocleidomastoi deep cervical flexors suboccipital, and trapezius muscles that reach your shoulders.

These muscles are crucial in the world of movement. They assist in supporting the neck of your shoulders, head and back. As with all muscles, the muscles of your neck are prone to injury and wear.

For the majority of people, shoulder and neck pain comes from strains, muscle sprains or tears. the reason for these injuries is usually result of overtraining, improper posture, or sports injuries.

Luckily, most injuries recover within a couple of weeks. However you must take care of the discomfort they result in. The way it usually works is when muscles get stretched to the point of being overextended small tears start to form within the connective tissues. These tears can cause pain, swelling, and can weaken your muscle.

The pain may be minor or severe. it could include shooting pains, tingling feelings as well as stiffness, numbness, spasms, or soreness. This can seriously hinder your day-to-day activities. The more severe the strain more severe, the more painful the inflammation will be, as well as the longer your recovery time. Even more the strain and sprain on your shoulder and neck muscles could cause you to develop knots, which can cause soreness and pain.

There are a few stretch exercises for your shoulders and neck that you can do to alleviate discomfort before it becomes worse. This includes:

Option 1:

Exercise one: Neck stretch for general purpose.

1. Place yourself in a comfortable place.

2. Begin to tilt your head slowly downwards until your chin is in contact with your chest. Keep this posture for approximately 5-10 minutes.

3. Lift your head gently back, and then raise it so that you're facing the ceiling. Keep this position for 5-10 seconds and then let go of the head by keeping your eyes straight ahead.

4. Relax your shoulders and slowly tilt your head towards your right side, as if you were striving to get your ears. Keep the head in this position for 5-10 seconds. Then, bring your head straight in front before tilting it back to your left until your eyes reach the same

position that your ear was previously was. Maintain the position for 5-10 minutes.

5. Take your shoulders off. Turn your head towards your left as if you were trying to see across your shoulder. Keep your head in this position for 5-10 seconds and then return to your starting position.

6. Move your head towards your left. It should be possible to see an object on the other side of your shoulders. Keep the posture for 5-10 minutes.

7. Let the position go and relax.

Exercise two Two: Neck back stretch

1. Take a step towards a wall and place your left hand towards the wall. Continue by raising your left arm then bend it towards the elbow, creating an angle that is right. Your palm should meet the wall while your hands should sit just above the top of your head.

2. Turn your head to the left, then gently bend it. You will feel a slight stretch in your neck as

well as your back. Take care not to overdo it and keep this stretch for 5-10 minutes.

3. Move to the other side with your left side towards the wall. Lift your right hand up and bend your left arm towards the elbow to create an angle of right angles.

4. Move your head towards the left and gently bend till you can feel a comfortable stretch. Do this for 5 to 10 minutes.

Exercise three Exercise three: Shoulder stretch

1. Straighten up with both your arms straight and bent at your elbows in order to form right angles. You can sit in the doorway to provide your hands with support while they are touching the door's frame from both sides.

2. Lean toward the forward. There should be a slight stretch under your collarbone. Keep it for 5-10 seconds.

3. Reverse gently back to the starting position.

When you're done with Exercise Three of the previous exercises, come back for Exercise One and do the exercise 3-4 times.

Option 2:

Exercise one Exercise one: Neck rotation

1. Straighten up or sit down on a chair that is firm.

2. Keep your chin in a straight line and slowly tilt your head to the right side. Maintain the position for between 15 and 30 minutes.

3. Move your head gently towards your left and then hold it for 15-30 seconds.

4. Repeat the exercise 2 to four times.

Exercise two: Neck stretch

1. Straighten up and keep your eyes directly towards the future.

2. Maintain your shoulder in the same position as you shift the right side of your ear toward the right shoulder.

3. Keep the position for approximately 15-30 seconds.

4. The left ear should be moved toward your left shoulder, without shifting your shoulder. Do this for 15 to 30 minutes.

5. Repeat the entire exercise up to 4 times.

Three exercises The third exercise is to stretch the neck forward.

1. Straighten up or sit straight on a solid chair.

2. Move your head to the side, but be careful not to put too much pressure on your neck.

3. Maintain the position for 15-30 seconds.

4. Repeat the exercise as many as four times.

Exercise four: Side stretch

1. Take two fingers off your right hand , and then proceed to make sure you touch the right side of your template.

2. Move your head to the right while you make use of your fingers to give resistance from the bend.

3. Keep the position for 6 seconds, and then return to the beginning position.

4. Repeat the exercise 8 to 10 times.

5. Put two fingers of your left hand onto the left side of your temple.

6. Turn your head toward your left side while you make use of your fingers to offer resistance.

7. Maintain the position for 6 seconds.

8. Repeat the exercise 8 to 10 times.

Exercise five Exercise five: Forward bend stretch

1. Straighten up and lie down straight on a sturdy chair.

2. Place your middle fingers and index fingers onto your forehead.

3. Lean forward your head as you employ your fingers to exert resistance in your opposite side.

4. Maintain the position for about six seconds.

5. Repeat the exercise 8 to 10 times.

Exercise six: Neutral position stretch

1. Put the hands of your left hand to the rear of your neck. They should be above your neck.

2. Retract your head while using your fingers to create resistance in your opposite side.

3. Make sure you count until six, and then take the position off.

4. Repeat the exercise 8 to 10 times.

Seventh exercise: Chin tuck

1. Take a towel and roll it up then lie down on the floor, and place the towel underneath your neck and ensure that your head is on the floor.

2. Begin to bring your chin into your chest. Make sure you don't move your head.

3. Then, count to six and take a break for 10 seconds.

4. Repeat the exercise 8 to 10 times.

When you are engaged in stretching exercises for your shoulders and neck to alleviate muscles pain, it is important to do it with care at every exercise. Keep in mind that the pain you experience comes from injured or overextended muscles. If you make a mistake and do not take care, you could aggravate the injury instead of addressing the problem.

Let's take a look at stretching exercises for muscles spasms.

The Neck and Shoulder stretch for Muscle spasms

Muscle spasms are as a result of muscle contractions and can occur at any time and at any time. When they occur in your shoulders and neck you might feel discomfort and tightness.

Muscle spasms can occur during the late at night. If they occur, you might awake suddenly at the end of the night. Or you could wake up with stiff neck or shoulder pain at the beginning of the day, and wonder which source of the pain. It could be because of:

* Bad posture

* Dehydration

* Strain due to exercise

* Stress from emotions

* Strapping a mobile around your neck

* Lifting large objects

* Carrying a large backpack on your shoulder

* Altering your sleeping position in the middle of the night

Poor posture while working on a computer.

* Repeated or extended neck movements, and

• Serious problems like whiplash, joint injuries and herniated disk

Exercises can be performed to relieve muscle spasms or significantly reduce their frequency.

Some effective exercises include:

1.

Exercise one Stretch neck

1. Get up or sit down in a comfortable position.

2. Grab your right hand and put it on top of your head.

3. Begin to lower your head with your hands gently. Make sure you are on the right side of your chest.

4. Keep your position couple of minutes before releasing.

5. Put your right hand over your head.

6. Utilize the left side of your hand and gently push your head toward the left side of your chest.

7. Maintain your position couple of minutes, and then return to the position you started from.

8. Repeat the circuit three times.

Exercise two: Scalene stretch

1. Get up straight and put two hands on your shoulders. Utilize the left side of your hand to gentlyhold your wrist on the left.

2. Utilizing your left arm, slowly draw your right arm and shoulder downwards while you move your head towards the left. This exercise will stretch the left side of your neck.

3. Once you've done that then apply the right side of your hand to secure your wrist to the left.

4. By using your hand to the right, slowly move your left arm upwards and shoulders back while you turn your head to the right side. This exercise will stretch your left side of your neck.

5. Repeat the exercise routine three times.

Exercise three Three: Neck lift

1. Place your feet on the mat.

2. Put your hands on your head like you're planning to sit-up.

3. Place your neck in your chest. Then, proceed to raise your head. Your shoulders must not be lifted off the floor.

4. Repeat the exercise five times.

2.

Exercise one Exercise one: Neck rotation

1. Make sure you are standing straight and your head to the right.

2. Begin to place your hands around the back of your head.

3. Simply pull your chin toward your chest. Then count up to 15.

4. Three times repeat the practice, and then release the exercise.

5. Straighten up and keep your head turned towards your left.

6. Begin to place your hands behind of your head.

7. Keep your chin in your chest and count up to fifteen.

8. Repeat the exercise three times.

Two exercises: Chin tuck

1. Straighten your body and place your hands on your chin.

2. Utilize your fingers to pull back against your chin in a way that you have double chin. Your eyes should be looking ahead even though your head is shifted forward.

3. Then, count to five and take the position off.

4. Repeat the exercise five times.

Threerd exercise: Scalene stretch

1. Place your feet in an upright position and then clasp both hands to your chest.

2. Begin to lower the left shoulder as you tilt your head to your right side.

3. Keep the position for between 15 and 30 seconds, and then return to the starting position.

4. Hold your hands in front of your back, then lower your right shoulder.

5. Place your head on your left side , and keep it there for 15-30 minutes.

6. Repeat the whole circuit three times.

Exercise four: Neck stretch

1. Straighten up and move your neck toward your right shoulder.

2. Make sure you hold your right hand and put it to the left side of your chin.

3. Use your palms to gently press your chin while looking over your shoulder. Then count up to 10.

4. Do the exercise three times.

5. Make sure you are standing straight and then tilt your head towards your left shoulder.

6. Make sure you hold your left palm in your hand and rest it onto the right side of your chin.

7. Make use of your left hand to gently press your chin upwards to gaze over your shoulder.

8. Start counting to ten, and then Repeat the process three times.

Exercise five: Scapular stretch

1. You can sit on a chair or stand straight.

2. Allow your hands to fall gently towards your sides.

3. Continue to pull your shoulders backwards, in a manner that you would like the shoulder blades be in contact.

4. Keep your position until you reach a period of five times and repeat the exercise two times until you have completed a set.

5. Repeat the 10 times.

Exercise six The stretch of the torso

1. Relax on a seat, then place your hands behind your head.

2. Move your head gently until you're looking at the ceiling.

3. Repeat the exercise 10 times, and then let go of the position.

4. Repeat the exercise throughout the day.

OPTION 3:

Exercise one The exercise is to raise the shoulders.

1. Stand or sit straight and then place your arms by your sides.

2. Make sure you have straight backs and straight, then straighten your back and raise your shoulders, without lifting your head.

3. Keep it for a few seconds.

4. Lower your shoulders back to your starting point.

5. Repeat the exercise 5 times.

Exercise two Exercise two: Shoulder rolls

1. Sit up or stand up straight.

2. Continue to begin rolling your shoulders. They will roll up, then back then back down.

3. Repeat the 10 times exercise, and then return to your starting position.

4. Your shoulders should be rolled to the other side. They should be rolled up, ahead, and then back down.

5. Repeat the exercise 10 times.

Exercise three Exercise three: Neck lift

1. Stand straight and straight.

2. Turn your head in a way that you were looking across your shoulder to the right. Don't lift your left shoulder or strain your neck.

3. Put your right hand on your head and pull downwards your head.

4. Keep the hold for 30 seconds, and then return to your starting position.

5. Your head should be tilted towards your left shoulder, but do not lift your right shoulder.

6. Put your left hand on your head and lower your head.

7. Keep it for 30 second, and then let it go.

Exercise four: Chin retraction

1. Sit straight or stand up. Your neck, spine, and head must be aligned.

2. Keep your chin up, but do not overdo it.

3. Bring your chin up and wrap it around your neck.

4. Repeat the exercise 10 times.

Exercise five The exercise five is to stretch the shoulders.

1. Your arms should be crossed at your chest.

2. Relax your shoulders like you're pulling your shoulders towards opposite sides.

3. Keep it for 30 seconds before releasing.

4. Repeat this exercise on the opposite side.

Exercise six Arm swing

1. Straighten your body and let your arms drop on your sides. Your palms should face towards your body.

2. While not lifting your shoulders begin to swing your arms upwards. Then, swing them upwards.

3. Lower your arms and then swing them backwards, without moving your body.

4. Continue the practice for one minute.

Exercise seven: Arm lifts

1. Make fists using your hands, then place your hands on top of your hips.

2. Inhale deeply while lifting your arms above your head. Your hands should be to your head.

3. Take the pose off and continue to repeat the pose 10 times.

Exercise eight: Forward bend

1. Make sure you are standing straight and with your feet separated. Your toes should point toward the forward direction and the distance between your feet should be longer than your hip distance.

2. Hold your hands in front of you and then blow your chest.

3. Utilize the muscles in your legs to keep the position. The knees must be bent slightly.

4. Move your arms slowly over your head slowly. Put your chin on your chest while your head is hanging down.

5. Maintain the position for 1 minute.

Exercise nine Pose of the Cat Cow

1. Your knees should be under your hips. Place your hands on your shoulders.

2. Take a deep breath as you gaze upwards.

3. Inhale slowly and bring your chin closer to your chest. Your spine should be extending towards the outside in a round form.

4. Do the exercise for a few minutes.

Tenth exercise Stretching the shoulder bent

1. Get down into the earth on four feet. Your knees should line up with your hips, and your hands should rest on your shoulders.

2. Take your right hand up and, with your palm facing upwards place it over your left hand.

3. Turn your head slowly towards your left side, while your weight is placed on your right shoulder.

4. Keep it for 30 seconds before releasing.

5. Repeat this exercise on the opposite side.

Exercise 11 Pose in reverse

1. Stand up or sit straight.

2. Connect your hand palms to your back. Your hands should be facing down.

3. Turn your hands so that your fingers are with their backs facing upwards. Your palms should face one the other.

4. Make sure you bend your elbows while you press your palms against each other and exhale out your chest.

5. Keep your back straight , and hold for 30 seconds.

Exercise 12: Cow face pose

1. Place your elbow on the back from your neck. Your palm should face downwards towards the spine.

2. Use your right hand to make use of the left hand to push your elbow toward your right side.

3. Keep it for one minute, then repeat the exercise on the other side.

Make sure to keep your body in a relaxed state while you work out. Let's examine ways to treat pain that is accompanied by headaches.

Chapter 2: Exercises For The Neck And Shoulder For Headaches

Have you ever thought that headaches could result from muscle spasms , or pressure in your neck? It's true. You will frequently feel tension in the neck area or lower back of the head. The headaches that you experience can be dull or painless. If they do occur the neck can feel stiff or swollen.

Many people prefer to relax until stiffness and soreness eases You can still do some exercises to help prevent further incidents. This includes:

1.

Exercise one Stretch neck

1. Stand or sit comfortably. The arms must be on your sides, with your shoulders at a comfortable level.

2. Make sure your right ear is pointing towards the shoulder to your left.

3. Let your left hand extend toward the floor, and continue to bend your fingers upwards.

4. Keep it for 30 seconds, then let go.

5. Repeat the exercise in the reverse direction.

Exercise two Exercise two: Seated fold

1. Place your feet on the floor and then raise your legs. You can rest in a blanket, or a a folded towel to support yourself if you need.

2. Lift your toes up and stretch your spine.

3. Bend towards the front with your hips. If you need to you need to bend your knees in order to become more comfortable.

4. Your forehead should be placed on your legs and then put your hands on your feet.

5. Keep the position for 30 seconds.

Exercise three Three: Child's pose

1. Place your knees on the floor, and then extend your knees to the side. Your heels should be resting on your buttocks. your big toes must be touching.

2. Put both hands over your hips, and extend your spine.

3. Reduce your torso to the level of your legs. Bring your hands forward and then place your face onto the floor. Relax your shoulders, arms and neck. Hold your position for 30 minutes.

Fourth exercise The needle should be threaded.

1. Get yourself on four feet. Your knees should lie hip-width apart and your hands should be spaced shoulder-width apart. Your feet's tops should be positioned on the mat and your spine should sit in a neutral place.

2. Put your right arm underneath your left arm, and then move your arms to the left side. Begin to lower your shoulder and ear toward the mat. Don't move your feet or knees.

3. For 30 seconds, hold the position for 30 seconds, before returning to standing on all fours.

4. Do the exercise with your opposite sides.

Exercise five: Dog that faces downwards

1. Get up on your feet on all fours. Your knees should be hip width apart, and your hands shoulder-width apart. Make sure you are able to relax your spine while keeping your spine in a neutral position.

2. Put your hands on the mat and place your toes in the mat.

3. Lift your hips upwards as you straighten the legs. Do not lock your knees.

4. The length of your spine will form an upside-down V when you lift your heels toward the floor.

5. Maintain this pose for 30 minutes.

2.

One exercise: Chin tuck

1. Make sure you sit tall and that your back is in contact with the back of your chair.

2. Bring your chin toward your throat, but do not turn your head.

3. Keep it for 5 seconds and then let go.

4. Repeat this exercise 10 times per hour to bring your shoulders, neck and head.

Exercise two upper trapezius stretch

1. Stand straight, or sit straight.

2. Slowly move your right ear towards your left shoulder, but do not move your shoulders.

3. Put your right hand on your left shoulder on the upper part of your head, then pull your head to your right side.

4. Maintain the position at least 30 seconds. You should feel a tug on your shoulders and neck.

5. Return to the beginning point.

6. Do the exercise from one side.

7. Repeat the exercise routine 2-3 times.

Exercise three: Stretching the Cat Cow

1. On all fours and make sure your wrists are between the shoulders, and your knees under the hips.

2. Release your spine into an upright position.

3. Inhale deeply and let your back arched. Then, lift your tailbone as well as your head.

4. Inhale as you lift your spine upwards toward the ceiling. Place your chin and tailbone in a tuck as you draw your abdominals toward your spine.

5. Repeat the entire exercise for one minute while you breathe in and exhale in the same manner.

Fourth exercise Head turns

1. Get straight.

2. Your head should be turned to the maximum extent it can be and then look at your right shoulder.

3. Ten seconds, hold for 10 seconds, before returning to the point where you started.

4. Make your head turn so far as it can take you and take a look at the left side of your shoulder.

5. Keep it for 10 seconds.

6. Repeat the exercise three times.

Exercise five: Scapular retraction

1. Sit straight or stand on your feet.

2. Take a moment to relax your shoulders.

3. Press your shoulders as if you would like them to meet.

4. Do the same exercise 10 times each time after each hour.

OPTION 3:

One exercise One: Upper trap stretch

1. Stand tall or sit straight, allowing your hand on the left to hang to your left side.

2. Put your right hand on your head, just over your left ear.

3. Utilize your hand and pull the head slowly toward the right shoulder. You should feel a slight stretch.

4. Keep it for 30 seconds, then return to the neutral position.

5. Let your right hand hang from your right side.

6. Put your left hand over your head, just over the right ear.

7. Bring your head towards the left side of your shoulder, until you feel an easy stretch

8. Keep it for 30 seconds.

9. Repeat the exercise circuit 2-3 times.

Exercise two Exercise two: Stretch the bow and arrow

1. Place your knees on the floor with them bent and your shoulders apart.

2. Continue to stretch your arms inwards. They should be in line with the floor. Your palms should be facing each other.

3. Your left elbow should be moved backwards like you're shooting an arrow or bow. Keep the lower part of your body.

4. Move your body to your left, and then pull your left arm as if you're twisting it.

5. For 10 seconds, hold the position and then let go.

6. Reach your arms forward.

7. Turn your right elbow inwards.

8. Move your body to your left and then slide your right arm backwards in a twist.

9. Keep it for 10 seconds.

10. Do 3 to 5 reps of the exercise for each side.

Three exercises: Chin tuck

1. Sit tall or stand up straight.

2. Move your chin toward your neck. Be careful not to move your head.

3. Keep it for 5 seconds.

4. Repeat the exercise between 3 and 5 times.

Exercise four: Neck extension

1. Stand straight and straight.

2. Simply tilt your head backwards until you are able to see the ceiling.

3. Keep the position for 5 seconds, then you return to your original position.

4. Repeat the sequence 5-10 times.

Exercise five exercise five

1. Stand straight, or sit up tall.

2. Begin to slowly lift your shoulders.

3. Your shoulders should be rolled back and downwards.

4. Repeat the exercise 5-6 times before returning to a neutral posture.

5. Begin to slowly lift your shoulders.

6. Your shoulders should be rolled up and down.

7. Repeat the exercise 5-6 times before letting it go.

Exercise six: Bridge pose

1. Set a mat on your floor and then lie down upon your back. Your arms should be by your sides, with your palms facing downwards.

2. Begin to bend your knees. Set your feet about hip width between each other on the floor.

3. Your feet and your palms should be pressed onto the mat as you raise your hips.

4. Inhale deeply , then lift your hips up.

5. Do this for 30 minutes. Keep your core muscles tight while you work out.

6. Begin to lower yourself slowly to the floor, then relax.

Seventh exercise: Wall stretch

1. Get up straight and let your back meet the wall. Set your heels in the direction of the wall that they reach. Make sure they be close to the wall, if they're able.

2. Spread both arms out against the wall to form the shape of a T.

3. Then, bend both of your elbows till they create 90-degree angles.

4. Move your arms upwards and downwards at the elbows.

5. Do at least three times the exercises 10 times.

The best thing about doing these exercises is that they can kill two birds in one fell swoop You can get rid of your headache, and try to remove the cause. However, always be mindful when performing the exercises.

Let's take a look at shoulder and neck stretching exercises for pain in the nerve.

Neck and Shoulder Stretches for Neck and Shoulder Stretches For

The pain of nerves can be debilitating and often manifests as a sharp pain that is accompanied by a burning feeling. It's usually like pins and needles have poked your. But, it can be more subtle and intermittent.

The type of pain you experience is because your nerves are suffering from inflammation or anatomical damage. If damage is caused and nerve roots are damaged, they become damaged or pinched and cause discomfort. The pain could radiate through your neck and shoulders into your hand or arm. It may also get worse when you do certain movements.

There are many exercises that you can do to ease the discomfort. This includes:

Option 1:

Exercise one side bent

1. Get up straight, then lift your hands and place them around your head.

2. Make sure your neck and head are straight. Then swing to the left and move to your left after which you will swing backwards from the waist. Make sure you don't move your body forward or forward.

3. Repeat the workout 10 times. If you'd like to boost the intensity of your exercise, you can make use of hand-held weights. Keep them in your head as you swing your upper part of your body left to right.

Exercise two Two: Shoulder shrug

1. Straighten your posture and begin to shake your shoulders back and forth throughout 30 seconds making sure that you are moving at a slow pace.

2. After the 30 minutes have expired Take a break for several minutes.

3. Move your shoulders forward and then up like you're looking to open your ears. Then, you move them back to the lower part before moving them backwards. Then continue to press your shoulder blades together.

4. Do the exercise for 30 seconds.

5. Repeat the process in reverse.

Exercise three Three: Child's pose

1. Relax your feet and place them on your heels. The feet's tops should be flat on the ground.

2. Lean slowly toward the side until your back is in touch with your legs.

3. Straighten your arms over your head. Your palms should be touching the floor.

4. Maintain your pose on for 30 second.

Exercise four Exercise four: Body twist

1. Place yourself on a sturdy chair. Be sure that you are straight with your spine and that your feet rest flat on the floor.

2. Put your left hand over your left knee, and continue to turn left.

3. Keep the hold for 5 seconds before returning to the beginning position.

4. Put your right hand at the the top of your right knee, and then proceed to turn to the right.

5. Maintain the pose for five minutes.

Exercise five: Neck tilts

1. Sit down or stand straight.

2. Then, tilt your chin towards your neck. It should be possible to feel the neck's back stretch.

3. Begin to slowly tilt your head upwards while looking towards the ceiling. Your chin should be lifted and down.

4. Repeat the exercise five to ten times.

Exercise six Head turn

1. Sit down or stand straight.

2. Make your face turn towards the right side like you're trying to glance over your shoulder.

3. Keep the pose for 5 minutes.

4. Return to the position from which you started.

5. Make sure you face your left, and hold it for five minutes.

6. Repeat the exercise routine 10 times.

Exercise seven: Median nerve slide

1. Relax on a comfortable chair.

2. Place your palm up in front of your face, and then proceed to examine your hand.

3. Lengthen your arm from the side, until your wrist falls below your shoulder. Your fingers should be pointed upwards. Be sure to keep your eyes on the motion of your hand.

4. Return to the neutral position.

5. Repeat the exercise on the opposite side.

Exercise eight: Prayer stretch

1. Straighten up.

2. Place your palms on the table as if you wish to pray. Your fingers should point upwards.

3. Lift your elbows even as you lower your wrists. Arms should remain in line with the floor.

4. Then slowly push your elbows to your right side as far as they will reach, then move them move them to your left side.

5. Ten times repeat.

Exercise nine: Towel slide

1. Use a towel to hold it close to your head.

2. Place the towel behind your back, and then make use of your other hand to grasp it near your lower back.

3. Continue to raise the towel as high as your hands will allow.

4. The towel should be pulled back with your thumb to the extent it can extend.

5. Continue to move your hands upwards and downwards for 30 seconds, and then let them go.

2.

First exercise Trapezius stretch

1. Place your feet on the floor and keep your spine straight.

2. Use your right hand to put it under your thigh.

3. Put your left hand on your head, and then use it to tilt your head to your left side.

4. Keep your pose on for 30 second.

5. Repeat this exercise in the opposite direction.

6. Repeat the exercise routine three times.

Two exercises: Chin tuck

1. Straighten up and sit down in a sturdy chair.

2. Put your fingers on your cheeks.

3. Make use of your fingers to pull your chin back to create double chins.

4. Keep your hands in place for 3 to 5 seconds , then let go.

5. Repeat the exercise between 3 and 5 times.

6. As you become more adept in chin tucks practice it with your hands.

Exercise three: Extend your chin Tuck

1. Continue to perform the chin tuck by taking your head off.

2. Move your head slowly backwards until you can see the ceiling.

3. Make a cheek tuck. then stretch.

4. Repeat the exercise two to five times.

Fourth exercise Head turn

1. Straighten up and look at the future.

2. Move your head slowly towards your left.

3. Maintain the posture for 5 to 10 seconds.

4. Slowly rotate your head left, and keep the head in the same place for 5 to 10 minutes.

Exercise five The exercise five is neck bent

1. Get straight.

2. Then, slowly lower your chin until your chest is at a level.

3. Take a break for a few seconds before returning to the original position.

4. Repeat the exercise five to ten times.

Exercise six Exercise six: Shoulder roll

1. Straighten up.

2. Continue to lift your shoulders and back, then down.

3. Repeat the process up to 5 times.

4. Do the exercise in the opposite direction.

OPTION 3:

One exercise: Trapezius stretch

1. Relax on a comfortable chair.

2. Grab your right hand and put it underneath the right leg.

3. Put your right hand over your head, and gently shift your head to the left.

4. Keep it for 30 seconds.

Exercise two: Posterior stretch

1. Use a towel to hold it in front of your head using both hands.

2. Take the towel and pull it in opposite directions, so that it will provide resistance when you turn your head forward.

3. Maintain the position for three minutes.

4. Do the exercise between 5 and 10 times.

Third exercise: Chin tuck

1. Your index finger should be placed finger on your cheek.

2. Utilize them to push your chin towards your neck.

3. For 3 seconds, hold the button.

Fourth exercise Head turn

1. Your neck should be straight and your shoulders must remain so that you straighten your head to the side.

2. Your head should be directed toward your right shoulder to see how far it will go.

3. Keep the position for 5-10 seconds , then return to a neutral posture.

4. Your head should be pointed toward to your right shoulder.

5. For 5 to 10 seconds before releasing.

Exercise five Exercise five: Shoulder roll

1. Sit up or stand straight.

2. Lift your shoulders up.

3. They will roll back, and then lower them.

4. Repeat the exercise 5-6 times.

5. Repeat the exercise reverse.

Exercise six Shake shoulders

1. Make sure you are standing straight and have your arms by your sides.

2. Slowly raise your shoulders and down, forming the form of a shrug.

3. Repeat the exercise for a few seconds.

While you do the exercises to relieve nerve pain, it is important to pay attention to your body's movements carefully as abrupt moves can cause nerve pain. Take your time and slow down the exercises if you feel intense pain.

Chapter 3: The Exercises For The Neck And Shoulder To Help Facet Joint Inflammation

Shoulder and neck pain can result from the loss of the facial joints. These joints are at which two vertebrae adjacent to the neck join. Injuries and arthritis are a major contributor to pain in the facet joint. The pain can be acute and painful. The discomfort gets worse when you press on joints.

This is why you might feel more pain when you get up in the morning, as the majority of people get up quickly after waking up. There is also the possibility of experiencing increased pain following prolonged periods of in a sedentary position. The pain can also extend to your shoulders and your upper back, creating additional discomfort.

You can try a few exercises to relieve the pain in your facet joints include:

1.

Exercise one Exercise one: Neck rotation

1. Sit tall and stare straight in the direction of.

2. Your head should be to your left and continue to go as fast as you can go but be careful not to cause it any further pain.

3. Focus your eyes at a spot on the wall . Hold it for 20 minutes.

4. Return to your start point.

5. Your head should be to you left side and move it to the maximum you is able to go.

6. For 20 seconds, hold the position before taking off the hold.

Second exercise: Forward stretch, and forward stretch

1. Stand up straight and focus your eyes on a point in the direction of your.

2. Begin to push your chin backwards until you have the appearance of a double the chin. There should be a feeling of stretching of your neck and your head.

3. For 5 seconds, hold the button.

4. Release the position and then return to the point where you started.

5. Reverse your head until you are able to comfortably gaze towards the ceiling.

6. Make sure to stretch for five minutes.

7. Repeat the exercise routine three times.

Exercise three Three: Neck stretch to the side

1. Stand up or sit straight.

2. Your head should be bent to your left. The left side of your ear must meet your left shoulder. However, it is best not to lift your shoulder until it touches your ears.

3. Begin to gaze up towards the ceiling. You'll feel a stretching in the back of your neck.

4. Maintain your pose indefinitely for twenty minutes before returning to a neutral pose.

5. Turn your head to your right. Your right ear should be in contact with that shoulder on your left. Do not lift the right arm.

6. Take a look up at your ceiling, and then hold this position for 20 seconds.

7. Relax.

Fourth exercise Trapezius stretch

1. Stand tall, or sit straight.

2. Move your head slowly towards your left. The left side of your ear must be in contact with to your right shoulder.

3. Then, you can move your chin to your chest. There will be a feeling of stretching in your shoulder and the neck's back.

Exercise five: Neck retraction

1. Place yourself in a chair and make sure that your spine and head are straight. Focus your gaze to a spot in the front of you.

2. Begin to pull your head back while keeping your shoulders in a neutral position. This should lead to you getting an upper chin that is double.

3. For a few seconds, hold and then let go.

4. Repeat the exercise five times.

2.

Exercise one Exercise one: Deep cervical flexor

1. Relax on your back and begin to lower your knees. Lay a towel rolled up on your neck.

2. Put your hand in a position and place it on top of your collarbone. This will allow you to observe any muscle movement that isn't yours as you stretch.

3. Move your jaw to relax and then your tongue towards the roof of your mouth.

4. Your chin should be moved towards your chest. Keep your head in a fixed position during the exercise. You must go as long as you can without feeling your muscles contract beneath your fingers that rest on your collarbone.

5. You should hold for 5 seconds when you're in the your position.

6. Release and return to your starting position. Be careful not to raise your head or press it back into the pillow.

7. Do two sets of the workout 10 times.

Second exercise: Isometric neck rotation

1. Sit straight or stand in a tall position. Put your chin into a tuck.

2. Your right thumb should be placed on your left cheekbone.

3. Make sure you move your head to look up at the right shoulder. Utilize your hand to resist the motion.

4. Tens the posture for 10 seconds before you let the pressure go.

5. Your left palm should be placed over the left cheekbone.

6. Move your head so that you look up at the left shoulder. Make use of your right hand stop the motion.

7. Keep your pose for 10 second.

8. Do 2 exercises 10 times in a row.

Three exercises Three: Neck side bend

1. Sit tall and stand up straight. Put your chin into.

2. Pick up your middle and index finger, and place them on the right side of your head.

3. Utilize your fingers to give resistance when you move your head the right.

4. Keep the pressure for 10 seconds Then release the pressure gradually.

5. Put your middle finger as well as your index finger to the left side of your scalp.

6. Make use of your fingers to provide resistance while you turn your head towards your left.

7. Ten seconds of pressure, and then release slowly.

8. Do two sets of the exercises 10 times.

Exercise four: Head rotation laying down

1. Relax on your back and put your head on the pillow. Bend your knees.

2. Move your head slowly towards your right side while exhaling. Be gentle with yourself.

3. Inhale and return your head to its middle. Rotate to the left when you exhale. Make sure that your movements are comfortable and painless.

4. Complete one set of the exercise six times.

Exercise five The upper trapezius Stretch

1. Straighten your body and sit in a relaxed posture.

2. Use your right hand to put on your lower back. This is where your back pocket is. Make sure to align your hands as easily as you can. Lower your shoulders.

3. Turn your head towards the left, then look down.

4. Place your left hand over your head and pull your head down further. Your neck should be feeling relaxed and shoulders stretch.

5. You should hold for 20-30 seconds.

6. Return to an upright position.

7. Your left hand should be behind your back, then lower your left shoulder.

8. Move your head towards your right side, and then look downwards.

9. Put your right hand on your head and lower your head.

10. Keep it for 20-30 seconds.

11. Complete two sets of this exercise and then let it go.

OPTION 3:

One exercise: Chin tuck

1. Relax on your back, then proceed to lower your knees. Your feet must be flat to the floor.

2. You should look up at the ceiling while you bring your head to your chest.

3. Do this for five minutes. You should feel a stretch in the top of your skull, all the way into your neck.

4. Repeat the exercise 10 times.

Exercise two Exercise two: Side to Side rotation

1. Lay on your back and gradually lower your knees. Make sure your feet are level in the air.

2. Begin to move your chin until it will be toward the right side of your shoulder. You can also utilize your hands to pull your head back further.

3. Make sure to hold the stretch for 20 minutes.

4. Make sure to move your chin as much as it is able to go towards the left side of your shoulder. Make use of your hands to offer an even more tense stretch.

5. Make sure to hold the stretch for 20 minutes.

6. Complete the exercise circuit up to 3 times, then, relax.

Exercise three: Side bend

1. Lay in a reclined position. Bend your knees and then place your feet to the ground.

2. Begin towards lowering your head to your left side. Right ear is supposed to lie close to the shoulder of your left. While you are doing the exercise, you should not move your shoulder. Instead, use your hand to bring your head back towards your shoulder.

3. Keep the hold for 20 seconds before returning to the neutral point.

4. Lower your head toward your left shoulder. Left ear is supposed to lie close to you left shoulder. Don't lift your shoulders. Use your hands to move your head closer to your shoulder.

5. Make sure to hold the stretch for 20 minutes.

6. Repeat the exercise routine 3 to five times.

Exercises can strengthen joints and muscles. They also alleviate shoulder and neck discomfort. But, you might not want to perform any exercise if you are already experiencing discomfort. This isn't a good idea. It is better to doing the exercises just a tiny small at a interval.

As you begin your journey with the exercises slowly in order to assess the body's response. In this way, if you're not hurting it is possible to perform an extended stretch. However, If you're experiencing discomfort, you should put off the exercise before you cause further injury to yourself. As you increase your endurance slowly, you'll relax your muscles and joints as time passes and in the end you'll be able perform complete stretch.

We will now take a look at shoulder and neck exercises to help with osteoporosis.

Chapter 4: Shoulder And Neck Stretches To Help Bone The Pain

Normally, the pain of neck comes from injury or disease on the tissues of soft tissue of the cervical spine. But, this doesn't mean that your bones can't be affected by pain. There is pain that can be felt within the vertebrae of your cervical spine. The pain can also be accompanied by some tenderness.

For relief from this pain, you may do exercises like:

1.

Exercise one Exercise one: Pendulums for shoulders

1. Sit near the counter or table.

2. Lean forward, without rounded back, and then place your left hand onto the table. The left hand should lie at your side and your knees shouldn't become locked.

3. Move your left arm gently from side-to-side and then make a circle 10 times.

4. Return to your beginning position.

5. Then lean back and rest your left arm upon the table. Put your right hand to your side.

6. Move your right arm gently from side to side , and then move it in circles 10 times.

7. Repeat the exercise again.

Exercise two: Crossover arm stretch

1. Relax your shoulders and stand straight. your shoulders.

2. Continue to drag you right arm over your chest as far as it will go while using your left hand to hold your upper arm.

3. For 30 seconds, hold the position and then let go.

4. Bring your left arm over your chest. Use the left hand secure your upper arm.

5. For 30 seconds, hold the button.

6. Repeat the exercise three times.

Exercise three Exercise three: Passive rotation

1. Make sure you have a cane that is lightweight or a stick.

2. Keep the stick in place using your right hand, then employ the left side of your hand tograsp the stick at the other side.

3. Begin in pulling your stick in a horizontal direction. You will feel a stretch the shoulders in front of you.

4. Keep it for 30 seconds, without bending to either side, or leaning to.

5. Switch hands and do the exercise again.

6. Repeat the exercise three times.

Exercise four Exercise four: External rotation

1. Find a cane or a stick that is lightweight.

2. Keep it in your right hand behind you, and then utilize the left side of your hand to cover the stick at the opposite end. Your stick must be vertical.

3. Make sure that your elbow is in the direction of your body. move the stick up and down.

4. Make sure to stretch until you've completed the stretch for 30 seconds.

5. Take a break to 30 seconds.

6. Take the stick in your left hand and then secure it by putting your right hand in the direction of your face.

7. Your left elbow should be at your side, begin to move the stick horizontally.

8. For 30 seconds, hold the position before letting it relax.

9. Repeat the exercise three times.

Fiveth exercise: Wall crawl

1. Make sure you stand straight on an object. Your fingers must be able reach the wall when you extend your arm.

2. Straighten your arm on the shoulder that is affected and continue using your fingers to walk across the wall in a slow, steady manner. Don't raise your shoulders or lean toward your ear.

3. Crawl to the highest point you can and hold it for 15-30 minutes.

4. Crawl back.

5. Repeat the exercise one or 3 times each time you attempt to get higher.

Sixth exercise: Wall push up

1. Standing straight on the wall. Make sure your arms are straight and then lay your hands flat against the wall.

2. Separate your feet until they are shoulder-width distance. Then, strengthen abdominal muscles.

3. Check that your feet are flat on the floor, then relax your chest while you move your elbows.

4. Slowly lower your upper body toward the wall. You'll be able to feel your shoulder blades come together in the back. Do this for 1 second.

5. With your hands on the wall flat As you pull your hands back, do so gradually until you can straighten.

6. Repeat the exercise 8 times.

7. Perform more repetitions of the exercise when you feel comfortable with the exercise.

2.

Exercise one Exercise one: Neck glide

1. Make sure you stand straight. Make sure you have straight neck.

2. Continue to move your chin back slowly.

3. Maintain the posture for 5 minutes. Return to the point where you started.

4. Do the exercise 10 times.

Exercise two: Neck extension

1. Get straight.

2. Slowly lower your head until you are looking upwards. Don't arch your back.

3. Keep your stretch for five seconds , come back into the neutral posture.

4. Begin to slowly move your neck to ensure that your neck is in your chest.

5. For 5 seconds, hold the position for 5 seconds, before returning to the beginning point.

Exercise three Exercise three: Neck rotation

1. Straighten up and look straight ahead.

2. Continue to turn your head left.

3. Keep the stretch on for 10 seconds before you return to the beginning position.

4. Your head should be towards your left.

5. Maintain this pose for 10 minutes return to your starting position.

6. Do the circuit exercise 10 times.

Exercise four: Lateral extension

1. Straighten up and look in the direction of.

2. Continue to lean toward your left side.

3. Make use of your left hand as resistance while you push your head towards the left.

4. You must hold for 5 seconds prior to you return to the beginning point.

5. Your head should be leaning towards your right side.

6. Make use of your left hand offer resistance when you push your head towards the right.

7. Keep the stretch in place for 5 seconds, then let it go.

8. Complete the exercise routine 10 times.

Exercise five Five: Shoulder shrugs

1. Make yourself stand up and stare at the sky straight in the direction of.

2. Lift your shoulders gently.

3. Keep the pose for 5 minutes.

4. Return to the beginning point.

5. Repeat the exercise 10 times.

Exercise six Sixth exercise: Forward flexion tilted

1. Get up and stand tall, and look straight in the direction of.

2. Continue to move your chin toward your left shoulder.

3. Then, turn your head downwards, and hold it for five seconds.

4. Return to the starting point.

5. Your chin should be pointing towards the right side of your shoulder.

6. Then tilt your head downwards, and hold it for 5 seconds.

7. Do this exercise every hour, if you work on the computer.

Seventh exercise Seventh exercise: Deep stretching

1. Letting your head rest on your back and allowing your head to rotate towards your right shoulder.

2. Utilize your left hand push your head further downwards. You can also use the opposite hand to secure the chair.

3. Keep it for 30 seconds.

4. Letting your head turn towards your left shoulder.

5. Make use of using your hands to move your head towards the ground.

6. For 30 seconds, hold the button.

7. Repeat the exercise routine three times.

Exercise eight: Resistance presses

1. Stand straight and sit tall. Your head should be in a neutral spot.

2. Put your right hand flatly on your forehead. Use it to apply pressure when you pull your head back. Make sure you don't tilt your neck.

3. Keep it for 5 seconds, then return to the beginning point.

4. Put your hands on the side of your head.

5. Begin to pull your head back by using your hands to create resistance. Make sure not to move your neck.

6. For 5 seconds, hold the position before letting it go.

Exercise nine: Towel pull

1. Grab a towel and place it in front of your neck. Your hands should hold the towel right behind your collarbone both sides.

2. Pay attention to the ceiling while you lay your head across the towel. Arms should be raised to help support your cervical spine while you stretch your head to the side.

3. Repeat the exercise 10 times , but without being in the same position.

The trick to do the exercises is to stop when you feel discomfort. If you can do this it is possible to keep doing the exercise or perhaps even do a more intense stretch. Keep in mind that the goal is to relieve pain rather than adding to the discomfort. Make use of your judgment to determine the distance you are able to get without causing harm to yourself.

Now let's take a take a look at shoulder and neck exercises to help relieve pain that is referred.

Stretches for Neck and Shoulder For Refused pain

Sometimes, pain doesn't start in your shoulders or neck. Instead, it originates from someplace else, and then moves to your shoulders or neck. This type of pain is referred to as "be referred" from organs like the heart or esophagus.

There are a few exercises you can perform to alleviate this kind of discomfort. But, it is recommended to consult a doctor when you're unable to determine the root of your shoulder or neck discomfort, to rule out the root reason.

The exercises comprise:

1.

Exercise one: Across your chest

1. Straighten up.

2. Continue to put your right arm over the chest.

3. Your left arm should be bent at the elbow, and then place your left hand over your right elbow, with your fingers spread.

4. Maintain the position for 1 minute.

5. Place your left arm across your chest.

6. Bend the right arm towards the elbow, and then place your right hand on top of your left elbow, giving it assistance.

7. Keep the position for one minute.

8. Repeat the exercise 3 to five times.

Exercise two Exercise two: Neck release

1. Get straight.

2. Continue to rotate your chin towards your chest. You will feel an increase in your neck.

3. Your head should be tilted towards your left.

4. Do the pose for 1 minute.

5. Move your chin downwards.

6. Your head should be tilted to the right.

7. Do the pose for 1 minute.

8. Repeat the exercise routine 3 to five times.

Exercise three Exercise three: Chest expansion

1. Straighten up.

2. Grab a towel or workout band. Use your hands to keep the band behind you.

3. Relax your chest while you bring your shoulder blades towards each other.

4. Tilt your chin upwards.

5. Keep it for 30 seconds.

6. Repeat the stretch between 3 and five times.

Exercise four The exercise four is: Spinal rolls

1. Stand tall and let your arms fall to your sides.

2. Make sure your elbows are crossed over your chest. The right hand should sit in the top.

3. Turn your elbows toward each opposite. Your forearms' backs should be in alignment

and your hands should extend until your palms are in contact.

4. Keep it for 15 seconds.

5. Inhale, and then twist your spine, bringing your elbows toward your chest.

6. Breathe in as you open your chest. Then, raise your arms.

7. Do the exercise for one minute.

8. Repeat the exercise in the reverse direction.

Exercise five Exercise five: Seated twist

1. Place yourself on the chair. The ankles of your feet should lie straight below your knees.

2. Begin to turn the upper portion of your body towards the right. The left arm should be moved towards your thigh.

3. Keep this pose for 30 minutes.

4. Repetition the same exercise for the right side.

5. Complete the exercise circuit three to five times.

Exercise six The exercises include shoulder circles

1. Straighten up.

2. Your left hand should be placed lightly against the seat, while your right hand rests on your side.

3. Continue to rotate your left hand in the circle five times and then move it five times in the opposite direction.

4. Switch hands, and then repeat.

5. Do the exercise two to three times a day.

Exercise seven: Shoulder stretch in the doorway

1. Place yourself in the entranceway. Your elbows and arms should create a 90-degree angle toward the ceiling.

2. Place your right foot to the front and then press your palms against the door frame.

3. Continue to lean forward until you work your core.

4. For 30 seconds, hold the button.

5. Put your left foot forward and continue the exercise.

6. Repeat the exercise circuit 2-3 times.

2.

Exercise one: Forward tilt and backward tilt

1. Sit tall and stand straight.

2. Continue to lower your chin toward your chest.

3. You should hold your head for between 15 and 30 seconds, then slowly raise your head.

4. Next, tilt your chin upwards. The top of your skull should rest on your back.

5. For 10 seconds, hold the position and then let it go slowly.

6. Repeat the exercise routine multiple times.

Exercise two: Side tilt

1. Get straight.

2. Be sure to gently move your head toward your right side, as it would be if you were

aiming to connect your shoulder to your ears. Do not lift your shoulders.

3. Maintain the pose for 5-10 seconds.

4. Do the exercises on your left.

5. Perform 10 repetitions of this exercise.

Exercise three Exercise three: Side rotation

1. Stand up or sit straight.

2. Your head should be pointing towards to your left shoulder. There should be a feeling of stretch along the sides of your neck and shoulder.

3. The pose should be held for 15-30 minutes and then release.

4. Make sure you are looking toward the left side of your shoulder.

5. For 15-30 seconds and then release.

6. Complete the exercise routine 10 times.

Exercise four Exercise four: Shoulder roll

1. Get straight.

2. Then lift your shoulders and then turn them around in a circular motion.

3. Repeat the exercise six times.

4. Take your shoulders up, and then turn them back in the form of a circle.

5. Repeat the exercise six times.

OPTION 3:

One exercise: Levator scapulae stretch

1. Sit straight or stand in a comfortable chair.

2. Turn your head to your left.

3. Turn your head towards your side in order to relax the neck muscles.

4. Maintain the position for 15-30 seconds before returning to the position you started from.

5. Make sure you tilt your head to the right then bend your head to the left.

6. You should hold for between 15 and 30 seconds.

7. Repeat the exercise 2 to four times.

Exercise two Two: Upper Trapezius Stretch

1. Sit in a comfortable chair or stand tall.

2. Relax your shoulders and secure yourself to the chair using your hands.

3. Your head should be moved towards your shoulder and keep it there for 15-30 seconds.

4. Return to the beginning point and then repeat the exercise on the other side.

5. Repeat the exercise routine 2 to four times.

Exercise three Three: Neck rotation

1. Get up and stand tall or sit on a sturdy chair.

2. Keep your chin at a level angle when you turn your face to the left.

3. Maintain the pose for between 15 and 30 seconds.

4. Turn your head to the left and continue to hold your pose for between 15 and 30 seconds.

5. Repeat the exercise routine 2 to four times.

Fourth exercise: Chin tuck

1. Place your feet on the floor, and then place an unrolled towel beneath your neck. Make sure your head is firmly on the floor.

2. Bring your chin down towards the neck's front.

3. Do the position for a period of six

4. Take 10 seconds to relax.

5. Repeat the exercise 8-10 times.

5. Forward Neck Flexion Exercise

1. Straighten up or sit on a comfortable chair

2. Begin in bending the head and hold it for 15-30 minutes.

3. Return to neutral.

4. Repeat the exercise two to four times.

It is important to keep in mind it is important to remember that even if you may not know what is causing your shoulder or neck discomfort does not mean that the pain will be any less. Pain that is not referred can hurt exactly the same as other kind of pain. This is why it is important to be extra cautious when performing exercises. Take your time and stop when you feel discomfort. So, you'll be able stop if you are uneasy.

Let's take a examine some suggestions to help you get relief from shoulders and neck pain at bay.

Chapter 5: Tips To Help Your Neck And Shoulder Reduce Pain

Exercises for the shoulder and neck aid in removing discomfort and restore your function. However, if wish to keep the pain at bay, you have to be more than just exercising. The root for the pain.

Here are some suggestions to help you get there:

Find a workplace that is suitable for you.

A large portion of workers spend up to 8 hours working each day. In this period, they remain in the same place for long periods of time, increasing the chance of injury. This is the reason you have to set up an ergonomic workplace. This kind of workplace is focused on your posture while you work. In order to create it:

Find a comfortable chair that allows you to put your feet flat on the ground while you sit

* Make sure that your knees are on an angle lower than your hips.

* Sit straight on your chair, keeping your arms positioned at an even level with the desk.

Make sure that your computer's monitor is level with your eyes.

* Put your keyboard and mouse close to your body so that you don't need to spread out when you make use of them.

When you've got a comfortable working environment, it is important to sit up at least every hour to stretch and eliminate the kinks off your body.

Be aware of your phone's habits

Consider the way you use your phone. If you get a message when your mobile rings turning your head downwards to glance at the message you received is simple. You can move your phone up to see the message, however, all this time your neck is tilting downwards. This puts constant stress on the neck muscles. To ease the strain

* Take your phone and put it on your eye prior to reading any messages. Don't tilt your head when you hold the phone.

Do not place phones between the ears and your shoulder when you are talking to it.

Make sure to use headphones or earbuds, and keep your neck in a straight position while you speak.

* Place your phone in a safe place at least every hour.

Stretch your muscles when you've finished using your phone. Relax your body.

It is also important to note that time can go through the air quickly when you use your mobile. This is why you may require setting alarms to keep track of your use.

Make sure you are in a good posture.

It is your posture that that you need to improve in order to prevent shoulder and neck discomfort. This is particularly important when you tend to slump your shoulders while relaxing and bend forward when working. When you are healing of pain must:

Be sure to stand correctly

When you stand up the head must be straight up with your shoulders straight, your chest inward with your hips locked into. Additionally, it will benefit if you were to distribute your weight evenly across both feet.

* Move around between now and the next time, rather than remaining in the same spot.

• Get a worktable that is standing and then raise it with one foot. You can rate it on an object. Change to the opposite leg after 5-15 minutes. This is the same for you are working at the kitchen.

It is important to stay away from sitting in the same place for extended periods of time. It is not advisable to avoid movement because of injury, but it is important to be patient and make sure you take frequent breaks to give your body a opportunity to recover.

Change the way you sit

Following injuries, the initial thing you should do is sit down for brief durations only. This means that you should stand for between 10 and 15 minutes. If you are sitting at a table, ensure that your hips and knees are at an angle that is right. You can utilize an ottoman or footrest to make sure you are at the right angle.

Put your feet flat on the floor , and try to avoid cross-legged exercise. Remember to also use back support. If you don't have a cushion you can comfortably sit on You can wrap a towel around your back and place it along the back's curve.

When you stand, step to the left so that you are sitting in edge on the side of the sea. After that you should straighten your legs when you stand instead of bent at your waist. After standing up Do 10 backbends standing up for stretching your back.

Stoop in fashion

If you're looking to grab something it is not a good idea to be bending your waist for it. If you do you'll end in straining your neck when you lower it down. Instead of bending at your waist it is possible to sit or kneel.

Then, find the object and then face it. Keep your feet in a slightly sloping position and gently lower yourself with your legs. If you need to lift something then bend your knees, and maintain the back straight. Avoid bending around the waist, and don't bend your neck in order to gaze towards the item. Instead, you should lower your gaze.

Be aware when you reach high above

Most people injure their shoulder and neck when they reach overhead to grab something off the highest shelf. This is particularly the case when the item they are reaching for is heavy.

To avoid injuries, make use of a chair or an exercise stool when you are reaching for something. Be sure to move near to the object and then use your fingers to raise it. It is important to be at the same level of what you're reaching to. If it's high it is possible to set it on a level surface prior to lifting it from the chair and lifting it up. When doing this, don't move your head. Use your hands to put the object.

Take care when driving

When driving, it's crucial to ensure you have back support. It is important to position it on the back's curve and ensure that your hips and knees are on exactly the same height. It is recommended to place your seat further away from the steering wheel, allowing your feet to be able to easily reach the pedals and you won't need to stretch out into awkward positions while you drive.

If you are planning an extended drive, plan for it in advance as you will need to take breaks between driving and this means that you need plan your route and determine the most appropriate places to stop for a break during your journey. It is also important to monitor your posture when driving. Depending on distance you'll need to set up several alarms that remind you to alter your posture if necessary.

Help create a peaceful sleep atmosphere

Sleep is essential as it gives your body time it requires to refuel and repair itself. If you're not in an ideal sleeping environment you could find yourself shifting and turning throughout the night and be awoken in pain when you put pressure on your shoulder, neck and back muscles.

To fix this problem, you should:

* Make use of a neck pillow When you put the pillow on your neck, ensure that it isn't too high. In fact, your head should naturally align with your body when resting on it.

* Purchase a more firm mattress Avoid one that sinks several places if you aren't looking to injure your body. Instead, choose a more comfortable mattress. It can initially feel uncomfortable however, your body will adjust and will thank you later.

Sleep on your back when recovering from an injury You should not sleep on your stomach or using an aid. Instead, you should sleep in a supine position.

Wear a mouthguard Some necks are injured due to the fact that they grind their teeth during sleep. If this is the case then you should invest in an oral guard.

Take a moment to relax before going to sleep - Sleep can be hard to find in the midst of a multitude of other things to do. This is why it is important to take a moment to relax prior to going to your bed. Set up a simple routine that lets your brain know that it's time to sleep.

Apart from creating a conducive atmosphere for sleep In addition, you must be cautious when you get up. You don't want to get up quickly or get up quickly when confronted with injuries.

Before getting up, lay on your back, and then pull your knees towards each other. Slowly move both legs back, and then utilize your hands to push yourself into a sitting posture. Get up, but don't lean forward in the waist.

Hydrate

Consider water in the same way you would think of a natural oil lubricant. You require it to lubricate your joints and muscles. However, many people don't drink enough water. To stop this from happening, be more mindful of the quantity of water you consume. For instance, you could set a goal to sip one or two glasses of this refreshing drink right after waking up.

It's also possible to decide to bring water every whenever you leave your home. The advantage of taking this approach is it makes you to drink plenty of water during the entire day. You can purchase a beautiful water bottle and then drink it throughout the day as time goes through. You can also add taste to the water with items like watermelon or cucumbers. In this way, if are not a fan of tasting water you could fool your brain to think you're drinking something different.

The goal is to drink at minimum 8 glasses water per day. Keep in mind that water is a source of nutrition for your body, and that includes joints and muscles.

Reduce stress

Stress is a wide range of signs, such as tension in the shoulders and neck. If you'd like to stay pain-free, then you must identify ways to ease stress. The things you can do to lessen stress include:

* Meditation: Meditation helps to heal the mind and improves your concentration. This helps you be less susceptible to stress and makes it easier to make better choices.

Music - Music can calm you in ways that other things aren't able to. The trick is listening to soothing music whenever you need to unwind. If you are listening to heartbreaking music, you might get caught in a cycle of soaking up the pain rather than let it go.

Find a passion It is a great way of changing your focus to more positive things. You can begin a activity like cycling or gardening to give yourself time to unwind. Your chosen activity must bring you satisfaction not a source of tension.

• Take time for yourself. Even if you can't take a vacation You should figure out ways to spend time with yourself. Take some time for yourself and inform everyone that they are not allowed to interrupt you during that period of time. Make use of that time to care for yourself.

In the end the way you carry out various tasks that you do in your everyday life can have a significant impact on your health and wellbeing. If you're looking to find an end to pain you must to be able to better treat your body.

Chapter 6: Signs And Symptoms

The condition of frozen shoulder is one which usually manifests with a series of. Each stage could last for a long time.

The freezing point is now attained. Every shoulder movement causes discomfort and the shoulder's range begins to decrease because of the pain.

The stage is frozen. In this time it's possible that the pain will start to ease. As time passes your shoulder will become stiffer, which makes it more difficult to move.

This is known as the thawing phase. The shoulder's range of motion is beginning to improve because of this procedure.

Certain patients experience more discomfort during the night, which could make it difficult to rest.

The Reasons

The capsule of connective tissues which surrounds the shoulder joint guards the bones, ligaments and tendons that form the joint. A frozen shoulder happens due to the fact that the capsule surrounding the shoulder joint expands and tightens, leading the joint to be restricted in its motion.

However, those who suffer from diabetes or those who were recently forced to put their shoulder in a sling for a long period of time, like following surgery or an injury to the arm are more likely to suffer from this complication according to medical professionals.

Risk factors that can increase

There is a chance that some situations can increase your risk of suffering from frozen shoulder.

Age and gender are crucial aspects to consider.

Women, particularly older than 40, are more susceptible than men to suffer from frozen shoulder.

Inmobility and decreased mobility are two distinct things.

If the shoulder is inactive or confined in movement for a long duration the likelihood of developing frozen shoulder is significantly increased. It can be due to many reasons, but are not only:

A damaged rotator Cuff

Arm is broken.

Stroke

After a surgery, it is essential to allow for a recovery time.

The body is affected by diseases that affect the whole body

Patients suffering from certain diseases are more likely to be at a higher risk of developing frozen shoulders. Conditions that could increase the risk of developing frozen shoulder include:

Diabetes

The thyroid gland is overactive (hyperthyroidism)

Thyroid that is not active (hypothyroidism)

The condition is known as cardiovascular. It's a condition which affects the heart and blood vessels.

Tuberculosis

Prevention

One of the primary causes of frozen shoulder is inactivity that may occur because of an injury to the shoulder or a broken arm or a period of recovery from stroke. If you've suffered injuries to the shoulder that has made the shoulder difficult to maneuver, speak to your physician about exercises you can do to maintain the motion of the shoulder joint once you've recovered.

Diagnosis

It's possible that your doctor may require for you to perform particular ways during your physical exam to assess your discomfort and determine the range you can move (active mobility). Then, your doctor might advise you to relax your muscles while they manipulate your arms (passive movement). The frozen shoulder affects both the active and passive ranges movement in the joint of your shoulder.

In certain situations the doctor might decide to administer a non-numbing drug (anesthesia) in your arm to determine your active and passive range of motion (ROM).

It is usually determined solely through symptoms and signs. However, your physician may recommend an imaging test like the X-ray or MRI to for you to rule out any other problems.

Treatment

The majority of the frozen shoulder treatments are geared towards easing shoulder pain while preserving as much motion as is possible in the shoulder.

Medicines

There are a variety of painkillers available for purchase like aspirin and Ibuprofen (Advil, Motrin IB, and many more) may help reduce the inflammation and pain that comes with frozen shoulder pain. Sometimes, your physician may prescribe stronger painkillers and anti-inflammatory medicines to ease your pain.

Therapy

It is possible to learn exercises for range of motion through a physical therapist which can aid in the restoration of as much flexibility within your shoulder as you can. It is essential to continue to perform these exercises to increase your recovery mobility.

Operative procedures as well as other methods

The majority of frozen shoulders will resolve in their own time, usually in between 12 and 18 months. If you experience persistent symptoms Your doctor might suggest these:

Injections of steroids. Corticosteroids in the shoulder can ease discomfort and help improve shoulder mobility particularly when the problem is in the beginning stages in the course of treatment.

The joints are stretched. To assist in stretching the tissues and making it easier to move the joint sterilized water can be injected into the joint capsule.

The manipulation of the shoulders. You'll be asleep and pain-free during the procedure as you'll have taken an general anesthesia. After the procedure is completed the doctor will then move the shoulder joint in different directions in order to help loosen the tissue that is constricted.

Surgery. Although the procedure on frozen or frozen shoulder joints is unusual, if no other treatment has been successful, your physician may recommend surgery to take out adhesions and scar tissue from the inside of the shoulder joint. The small incisions around your joint are made by your physician and then illuminated, tubular tools are inserted in the joint (arthroscopically).

Healthy home remedies and a lifestyle

Keep using the affected shoulder and the extremities to the maximum extent possible regardless of discomfort or limitations in range of motion. Applying ice or heat to your shoulder may help ease inflammation and pain.

Alternative medicine is a term used to describe a treatment that describes a medical practice that isn't conventional.

Acupuncture

Acupuncture refers to the incision of needles with a thin diameter through your skin at specific areas of your body to relieve discomfort. In most cases the needles remain there for anywhere from 15 to 40 minutes. It is possible for them to be moved or altered in that time. Because the needles are thin and flexible, and because they are usually placed in a superficial manner most acupuncture sessions are painful.

Transcutaneous electrical nerve stimulation (TENS)

Transcutaneous electric nerve stimulation (TENS) device provides small amounts of electrical energy at specific points along a neural path. When it is administered via electrodes that are taped to your skin it is not hazardous or uncomfortable. While we don't know what TENS does however, it is believed that it could stimulate creation of anti-pain chemicals (endorphins) or could inhibit pain fibers that transmit signals of pain to ease discomfort.

You're getting ready for your appointment.

When you first talk with your primary physician and ask them to suggest you see an orthopedic doctor who is trained in orthopedics, if your particular condition justifies it.

What can you do to assist

You might want to prepare a an inventory of the following things before you go to the appointment:

Please give specific details about the symptoms you are experiencing.

The information you need about health issues you've encountered in the past

Information about medical conditions your siblings or parents are suffering from.

The medicines and nutritional supplements you're taking now

Questions to discuss with your doctor

What exactly can you expect from your doctor

A few of the following questions can get asked of your physician:

What was the first time your symptoms began to appear?

Do you have any habit that causes your issues to get worse?

Have you ever experienced problems with your shoulder?

Do you suffer from diabetes?

Could it be that you've recently had surgery or have you experienced a restricted shoulder movement?

The Treatments for Frozen Shoulder are Secure and Effective

A frozen shoulder can be extremely painful. Some doctors decide to treat it by using hormones (such corticosteroids) and numbing drugs or painkillers, and in some cases the use of arthroscopic surgery to loosen the joint capsule, which is swelling. If the pain becomes unbearable, it is possible to take an over-the counter pain reliever (such as Ibuprofen) to ease your recovery and resume your normal routine as quickly as you can. Most important to keep in mind is to focus on addressing the root of the issue in order to stop suffering from becoming chronic.

A natural approach of frozen shoulder pain is to focus to gradually increase the range of motion with the application of focused and safe exercises that extend the shoulder using natural painkillers and reducing inflammation

1. Apply heat and stretch the shoulder joint.

It is important to warm up your shoulder prior to starting shoulder exercises to treat frozen shoulder is vital for increasing blood circulation in the affected region and to prevent further injuries. When dealing with a frozen shoulder, patience is the key therefore, allow ample healing time and to move slowly. The goal is to gradually gently, slowly, and carefully return movement to the shoulder. However, this could take time so don't rush things.

In terms of stretching and warming the shoulder, the most effective strategies are applying the heat for 10 to 15 minutes, having an ice-cold shower or bath (particularly one that has Epsom salt) and then starting to gently move your shoulder in small circular movements as much as is possible. You can either create your own heat pad or buy an expert heating pad for this use.

It is crucial to focus on any minor stiffness or tightness when stretching the shoulder to ensure that you don't overextension yourself too rapidly. One method of assessing the severity is to observe the pain after stretching. It should ease within 15 minutes, if done properly. Be sure to let your muscles to relax so you're performed onto soft tissues (rather than rigid and rigid) throughout the stretch. In order to gradually increase your range of motion as well as flexibility of your tight shoulder, you should consider taking your time when performing any of these simple shoulder stretches and exercises for 2 to 3 times a day for a start to ease your pain.

Experiment with rotating your arm outside by opening and closing the door or cabinet while you lie down and lift your arms straight over you.

Place your feet on the floor and create the "T" shape using your arms by stretching their arms outwards and touching the floor.

2. The Shoulder Muscle Exercises Feel More Improved

Researchers from Harvard Medical School recommend that you try the following set of exercises for your arm or shoulder as described below following warming up the stiff shoulder. Ensure that you're at peace (deep breathing can aid in this). 5. Move your shoulder and stretch it until you feel a moderate strain, but stop when you feel any discomfort. In the initial couple of weeks, concentrate on increasing you flexibility as well as mobility. Then, you can add resistance exercises for your shoulders to improve the strength of your shoulder.

Pendulum stretching Relax your shoulders, then sit up, allowing your affected arm to hang downwards. Begin by circling the arm around 10 times per direction, starting from the elbow. Repeat this every day for the first time and gradually decrease the frequency as you experience stiffness. Increase the amount of repetitions or do several sets every day. You can also try to gradually increase the length of your arm's movement by adding a tiny quantity of mass (for instance, putting three to five pounds of dumbbell in your hands). This will help free the shoulder joint further.

Take one side of a smaller towel (approximately three feet in length) within your hands and then draw the towel to your back and hold the other end by using your hand. Moving your upper arm upwards helps to stretch your shoulders. At the same time, pulling the opposite arm downwards helps strengthen your arms. Do this stretching between 10 and 20 times per every day.

Retract your steps and put your hands to the walls at waist-level with your arms slightly bent in the front of the wall. In order to stretch your arm as high as you feel comfortable and then slowly move your fingers towards the wall. Repeat the exercise starting every 10-20 times per day, beginning at the beginning.

Cross-body reach: With your arm that is healthy and a strained arm, lift your arm at the elbow, and then pull it back and over your body to ensure that you are able to hold an extended stretch across your entire arm for about 15 to 20 seconds. Then repeat the procedure. Try to reach farther throughout your body as your flexibility improves. Repeat this workout 10-20 times a every day.

Place the arm affected on a table which is about breast-high, and then extend the armpit (a counter-top can be a good spot to exercise). Slowly straighten and bend your knees to widen the armpit. Then, go into the squat position and bend a little more deeply each time, about 20 times per day to ease tension in your armpit muscles.

The rotation can be done in two directions This exercises for strengthening and rotation require more resistance. They is recommended when mobility and discomfort have been improved and discomfort has diminished. Be sure to warm up by stretching the arm which is being affected first. Use a rubber exercise band between your hands and rotate the lower part of the affected arm upwards for 15 to 20 seconds. This will allow you to develop outward rotation and strengthen. If you are looking to increase your rotation inwards take the other the ends of an workout band around a doorknob , and pull the band towards your body for 15 to 20 times per every day.

The physical therapy option is the 3rd option.

But, even though the exercises listed above are easy enough to do on your own, if you feel that pain persists and causes difficulty to move about or complete regular tasks, you should consult physical therapists who will suggest specific exercises and stretches that aid in improving your flexibility, range of motion and flexibility. Some patients need 4 to 12 weeks of rehabilitation in order to recover from freezing surgery and after that the range of movement generally is restored to normal. In some cases, it could require longer.

4. Natural Methods for Numbing Pain

You've likely already learned the best way to treat frozen shoulder is moving your shoulder gently and slowly. On contrary, could cause pain and discomfort. Alternatives to medicines include essential oils and other relaxants, are able to ease pain with holistic home remedies for frozen shoulder.

In order to increase circulation, reduce inflammation, and ease pain in your shoulder, apply peppermint oil onto it.

5. Reduce Inflammation and prevent complications from occurring

Spending time on an energizing diet and taking anti-inflammatory supplements to assist in healing can aid in reducing inflammation in the long term and help keep injuries from becoming recurring. Turmeric as well as omega-3 fatty acids, magnesium and CoQ10 are a few anti-inflammatory botanicals and vitamins that are available.

Many different types of fresh vegetables and fruit, probiotic-rich foods (yogurt, kombucha, kefir, and cultured vegetables), grass-fed beef, wild-caught fish, cage-free eggs, and healthy fats such as nuts, seeds, avocado, coconut oil, and olive oil are all good sources of inflammation-fighting nutrients. Make an effort to reduce exposure to other factors that can cause inflammation, like the stress of your mind and being overweight or obese, sitting for prolonged durations, smoking cigarettes smoke, chemicals or toxic exposure, as well as excessive levels of vibration exposure from vehicles (for instance, being truck drivers to earn money).

Exercises to stretch the shoulders

If additional areas of stiffness are identified the muscles can be stretched with the same technique. One of the main techniques for stretching is to help the muscles relax so that the stretch can be delivered to your soft tissues, without being interfered by muscles. The muscles in the shoulder are sensitive to being stretched abruptly and forcefully, or with the force of a lot Therefore, avoid doing it. In the end the aim is to give a gentle stretch to ensure that discomfort is reduced to a minimal. After the exercises Any discomfort should diminish after 15 minutes.

The shoulder stretching routine is recommended to be done at least three times per daily by the user. If it is possible, these exercises should be performed after the shoulder is relaxed, for example through hot bath or shower or participating in an aerobic exercise. Keep track of the most range of motion that you can achieve with each each stretch. After you've completed them attempt to establish an additional "bench mark" every time you finish the exercises to keep track of your progress as time passes.

The great thing about this method of training is that you're fully in control of the circumstance. You can alter the intensity of stretching to get the results your shoulder can handle the most easily. The program is mobile, and is able to be performed at any time, whether it's your office, home or vehicle, train, bus or any other place in which you are. It is crucial to keep regularity in this exercise routine will pay dividends. If you feel uncomfortable as a due to your exercise regimen, do not cut back or alter the intensity of your workouts. Instead decrease the intensity of your stretches until you feel comfortable.

Regular exercise can help keep your joints flexible and keeps the joints from stiffening. An hour of aerobic exercise every day is suggested to increase the "lubricating" impact on joints.

There are many kinds of fitness workouts.

You can get the exercise you need in a variety of ways, like running or walking, using an electric or stationary bicycle or running, climbing stairs or using a cross-country ski simulator, for instance. If you're unsure about your capability to perform this kind of exercise routine be sure to talk to your primary health care provider. Alongside exercising regularly, it's essential to devote an hour or so of your time to a cardiovascular exercise in addition to the stretching routine. For up to 30 minutes at a heart rate that is two-thirds of your maximum heart rate is suggested for those who have an active lung, heart, and blood pressure, as per the recommendations. The maximum heart rate you can achieve is determined by subtracting the age of 220 from your total and then dividing the results by 2. It is suggested that you consult your physician prior to starting this part of your program, particularly when you are older than 35 and haven't been active for a long time, or if you are uncertain about your fitness level.

The fact that some patients have "had treatment" can make them reluctant to take part in this aerobic and stretching program. We've had the observation that a lot of people who haven't responded to treatment in a formal manner are able to improve their shoulder strength by following the guidelines in our home exercise routine. Remember that the pain in your shoulder is persistent over an extended period of time. It's possible that improvement in your range of motion and ease is not likely until six weeks of regular involvement in the program. It is important to continue doing the exercises till your shoulder has regained the normal movement range and feels relaxed and comfortable.

We have found that medication isn't particularly effective for treating tight shoulders. This treatment regimen can be utilized together with moderate analgesics (such as ibuprofen or aspirin) when the patient wishes to use them. Patients have told us that narcotic drugs, "muscle relaxants," and sleeping pills haven't proved to be beneficial.

It's possible that you'll be able to use your shoulder in your comfortable zone. You ought to try certain water exercises or swim in the event that you are able to do it without damaging your shoulder. Exercises that cause pain in the shoulder On the other hand must avoid at all times.

Chapter 7: Cause Of Shoulder Tendon Problems

There is no joint in our body that is as intricate as the shoulder. Therefore, first of all, let me briefly discuss the shoulder.

The shoulder is often thought of as a ball joint made of head of the humerus, which sits inside the space. But, it is just one of of 5 (!) joints that make up our shoulder.

Our shoulder functions only by the precise timing between our head of humerus as well as the blade of our shoulders. Additionally the purpose of the shoulder blade is performed through the correct mechanics of the thoracic spine. Therefore, any method that doesn't take into account these three aspects at a larger level is doomed to fail!

In a nutshell the components create an object that is similar to the awe-inspiring precision of the clock mechanism. However the more complicated an item has become, the higher susceptible it is vulnerable to errors. Any neural or structural imbalance within this structure could manifest its self in the form of a dysfunctional shoulder function.

Our tendons are also a component of this system and perform a vital function as a strength transmitter. They are the ones that suffer when excessive stress can be induced to a poorly functioning joint. This can happen through sports or from everyday activities of the shoulder, for instance when your shoulder is in active use.

When our tendons become worn and tear, our bodies activate inflammatory mechanisms to begin repair of the tissue. The inflammatory process also makes the tendon tissue thicker, which can result in an even greater wear on the tissue. In this situation there is a feeling of "jumping" within the shoulders as we rotate the shoulder.

Then, in the most rare cases , the regeneration of tendon goes on without issue. As the process progresses it may lead to scarring and the growth of nerve endings and blood vessels.

The result is that a chronic tendonitis can quickly become a long-term issue.

Tendon tissue tissue that has a low circulation (bradytrophs) this is why convalescence tends to be longer in the case of such issues. However, the methods included in this book must be aimed at bringing about recovery of your condition as fast as is possible.

Cortisone isn't always an ideal choice

Doctors are not always equipped to deal with wear-related diseases. Today, a lot of orthopedics and physicians do not understand the meaning of wear marks as it occurs in a tendon problem.

Instead, they apply an approach that targets traumatizing situations and, in the end, result in inadequate outcomes. In these situations the most common approach is to treat the wear marks using antiphlogistics, such as the consumption of oral anti-inflammatory drugs such as Ibuprofen in high doses or cortisone injections into the tissue affected.

It is often overlooked that inflammation is only present at the beginning of the tendon diseases. It is the process of progressing and is described as degenerative and an inflammation-related disease!

In the initial inflammation the body is attempting to begin the process of regeneration of the tissue that has been damaged. In the meantime, it was demonstrated by studies that the suppression of an inflammation process is counterproductive and impacts the recovery of tendon structures.

Cortisone also comes with the ability to continuously damage its tendon structures, something that must not be the aim of a degenerative condition.

I'm not saying that cortisone injections are not appropriate in every situation however the usage of anti-inflammatory drugs for tendon injuries is something that must be considered thoroughly.

For the physician, treatment of an anti-inflammatory drug is the most effective method to ease the patient for a short period of time. However, the odds that the issue are very high after the effective use of anti-inflammatory drugs because the symptom was treated, it was not the reason for the issue.

The method presented in this book addresses the root of the issue and is intended to bring about an indefinite relief from suffering.

Modification to your current training program

This chapter will be particularly relevant to users who have completed an exercise program. Here are some guidelines to think about in order to become free of pain.

Be sure to avoid everything that can hurt!

This should be the primary rule to follow when choosing your workouts. The training that is difficult is only advised in certain circumstances and under the guidance by an expert. If you don't have any other guidance, this is the only suggestion to be following!

The problem becomes more severe as you progress through each training session without or in pain and the length of convalescence is unevenly increased most of the time. This is why I advise taking the appropriate steps when shoulder pain is first noticed.

Get a proper warm-up

It is important to do a re-mobilization of your shoulder prior to each exercise. To do this, you could utilize the exercises included that are in the book. It is important to not start immediately using your weights during the initial set of the exercises for strength. In the long term an effective warm-up is among the most beneficial practices you can make for your shoulders as well as the rest of your joints.

Beware of overhead movements

The most common approach is to focus on the motions that are above your head. Particularly, tension above the head motions caused by incorrect shoulder mechanics need advised to avoid! Above the head the shoulder is in a difficult position and the consequences of the tendon structure could be more evident due to an improper shoulder mechanic.

Pulling motions are preferred over pushing motions

The motions of pulling are typically more comfortable for your shoulder in comparison to push motions. Also, you can strengthen the muscles that straighten by pulling motions. This is very beneficial to a proper shoulder mechanic. For long-term shoulder health your exercise routine should be based on pushing and pulling motions at the ratio of 2:1.

Change to an unidirectional grip

A neutral grip that has your palms facing one another is preferred over an upper grip since it allows for more space within the joint of your shoulder. If you are required to modify your exercises according to that direction.

Begin to work closer to the body

The more closely you hold your hands close to the body, the more comfortable the workout will be towards your shoulder. When you are doing the motions of pulling and pushing make sure you select a posture for your shoulder that allows your arms to be as close as they can to your body.

Do not do anything that causes pain!

Oh, did I already say that?

I'll repeat it!

Problems with nutrition and tendon health

The subject of nutrition isn't the first one that is thought of when you think of shoulder issues.

But, your diet has more of an impact on this condition than you imagine. Certain foods may increase the degree of inflammation within your body, which can, in turn makes it more difficult for your body to manage the repair of the tendon structures.

The results of the mentioned measures vary for each individual. If you are able to see an improvement in shoulder pain, you should do everything you can to make it happen. If you do not see improvements in 30 days, you should contemplate whether to return to the old diet.

Remove all wheat products from your diet plan

A lot of people have a low tolerance to the protein in that grain (gluten). Even if there aren't any direct consequences of eating wheat, it's a good idea eliminating wheat from your nutrition program for testing reasons. If you have a lower tolerance to gluten, it can damage the intestinal wall, which can cause an increase in the inflammation factor within the body. Noodles, in addition include wheat products.

Take all milk products off your food list

Similar to the case of gluten, it also applies to any type of dairy product. In this case, it's the casein protein that cannot be processed in a similar way by all organism. Therefore, it is suggested to eliminate milk-based products.

Choose to eat vegetables instead of processed food items

Your diet should consist mainly of foods that are not processed, like various vegetables. High blood sugar levels due to processed food trigger inflammation. Also, ensure that your body is getting enough protein, which is 1g per kg of body weight. Protein can be derived through meat, fish or plant protein sources.

Supplemented Cissus Quadrangularis

The plant has been utilized for centuries in Indian medical system and has proved to be effective, particularly against tendon and joint problems. While the common joint supplements such as the glucosamine and chondroitin have an insignificant effect on tendon injuries in the best scenario, you will find several positive feedback from users of the Cissus extract.

An insider's secret!

Recommended dosage: 3g / day

Supplemented omega-3-fatty acids

If you consume a small portion of seafood, taking omega-3-fatty acids that are found in forms of capsules with salmon oil is definitely worth it. They may aid in the reduction of inflammation levels and have a positive impact on joint discomforts.

Dosage recommended: 3-5 grams daily of fish oil

The recommended supplements by me are available in the reference section in this book.

The program

Are you curious about the most common reason why people fail in a program that works?

They don't stay with it! Better yet they don't stay with it for long enough.

This is why I've designed a program that is suited to your lifestyle as closely as feasible. Only when you are able to apply the principles of the program on a regular basis over 30 to 60 days, you will see improvements!

If you're searching for an immediate solutions, you'll find nothing!

This program requires seven minutes each day, and every night. I've consciously created it so that every program is a set time for you, similar to the regular brushing of your teeth.

Think about the your quality of life is costing you right now.

Then, is 14 minutes per day to ask?

The created time specifications indicate the minimum amount of time you should devote each day. If you plan to take more time to achieve faster results. The morning/evening routine is only one of the ways to incorporate the workout in your daily life. It's not a issue if you wish to switch to a different routine.

The program comprises the following elements:

Morning Routine

Breathing

- Fascia Therapy

- Mobilization

Evening Routine

- Muscle Strengthening

Stretching

- Voodoo Floss

Each of these parts is important, and I would advise you to avoid the content when you are unable to perform them due to discomfort. If you are able to complete your homework every day and you are diligent, you stand a great chance of finding a solution to your issue.

What equipment is required?

In order to implement the program, you'll need equipment that you don't have.

Think about these factors before you become angry about the costs for follow-up:

The product is not much and is the most effective option to invest to improve your well-being! It is much less than the cost of an hour of physiotherapy, and will last for years!

You can buy similar products all over the world, but you'll locate the recommended products listed in the resources list at the end of this book.

Gymnastic Ball

The ball for gymnastics is useful for your training. When it's not being used, it could also be used to serve as an seating space.

Lacrosse Ball Set

You'll need a minimum of three lacrosse balls to accomplish the treatment of your tissues as well as for the purposes of mobilization. Two of them are connected to one another using tape. They are used primarily to treat the cervical spine. I'll explain how they work in the chapter "mobilization". The remaining ball is utilized to perform treatment of the tissues. Further details on this are in the Chapter "Fascia Therapy".

Foam Roller

Foam rollers are the ideal all-rounder for athletes. It is able to treat nearly every body part by using it. There ought to be a few of them in each sports bag.

Voodoo Floss Band

The voodoo band is possibly the most skewed one among the tools listed. It's not in the market for time, yet it is essential to the regrowth of your tendon! Even though the treatment isn't without pain After just one application, you'll notice an improvement.

The benefits of the voodoo floss are different. It is able to achieve a quick reduction of muscle tension. It also works on your tissues and fills the area of treatment with blood. If you've never had prior experience with the voodoo floss it could seem odd and uncomfortable to you initially. Do it nevertheless. The marks that could be left are gone next day.

We now move on to the various components that comprise the entire program!

Part 1 of the Program Part 1: Breathing

The first step to lead the way to success for you is breathing. It is better to use the right breathing! Your breathing is directly related to the shoulder issue.

Let's suppose that poor breathing could cause shoulder pain and we take an average of 17.280 breaths per day. Shouldn't it be an obvious consequence that the risk of developing shoulder pain is excessive due to breathing problems caused by improper breathing?

So far, you'll be able to agree with me! But you're still not certain of the way in which your breathing pattern is connected to the shoulder issue.

I understand! But there's a clear explanation!

The way we breathe is generally dependent on our own willpower. However, it can be affected by external influences such as pain, stress or anxiety.

If the influencing factors persist for a longer period of time such as for an overly stressed person improper breathing may be a routine.

We are aware of how effective the breath is not later than when we think about the cycle from a different perspective.

Deep, conscious breathing practice is believed to help us relax, reduce the heart rate, and increase Alpha waves within our brain. This demonstrates how crucial good breathing is to our bodies.

The incorrect breathing is often associated with an incorrect position, movement and the activation of muscles. Then, at the point, breathing pattern in relation to your shoulder pain is fascinating!

In the midst of our daily lives we are often able to develop breathing that occurs in the upper region of the thorax.

In this sense we frequently refer to "shallow" breaths. The diaphragm was designed to raise up and down with each breath. However, the proper usage of the diaphragm not anymore accompanied by superficial shouting!

The body is supported by additional muscles while breathing, referred to as extra respiratory muscles. But, when you breathe shallowly, your body triggers muscles that aren't designed to serve as respiratory accessory muscles.

Have you ever returned home from a long and tiring day at work and you felt your neck was tight and tight?

This is a great illustration for the above scenario and, in addition it is possible to link it with an insufficient activation of the muscle during the process of breathing.

However, tensions aren't the only result of working in a busy environment. The overactive muscles of your upper trapezius create a tension on your shoulder blade , and consequently, is a significant part of the function of the shoulder girdle!

If the muscle is tight and the pull becomes too large, an imbalance in shoulder mechanics develops. This is why permanent, wrong breathing can result in shoulder pain.

Every exercise begins with 20 proper breaths. They are the foundation for any further exercises! It is also important to begin observing your breathing throughout your daily day.

1. Exercise: Crocodile Breathing

Place your body flat on your back. The one hand is resting on your stomach while the other rests on your the thorax. Your neck and shoulders are in a relaxed state.

Then, take an inhale into your nostrils. While doing this your abdominal wall beneath your palm should raise, however, not your thorax! Try closing your eyes and trying to allow your breathing to become as slow and deep as it is possible.

Fascia Therapy

In the second section of the program we will focus on our soft tissue.

This portion of the programme is among the most crucial aspects of the program and must be included in any rehabilitation program.

If the words fascia, soft tissue, or SMR (Self Myofascial Release) do not sound familiar I'll quickly clarify them for you.

Your muscles, bones, tendon and all other types of tissue within the body is covered in connective tissue, also known as fascia. If the fascia is left in the same place for longer durations or is exposed to stress frequently, it will store selectively collagen, and the fascia becomes "sticky". Because collagen stores are stored, your tissue's quality decreases and the tissue will not function as it was intended to.

Perhaps you've had a treatment performed by a physiotherapist prior to.

The most common method employed by the physiotherapist involves streaking your tissues under pressure. In addition, this is how he can dissipate the collagen adherence that is already present and reduces the muscle tension.

In some cases, there is no need for the services of a physical therapist. However, in some cases it is better by doing things on a regular basis instead of waiting for our next appointment.

A single measure is as an immediate success like the work on the soft tissues!

The pain you feel during specific exercises are a sign of the condition that is present in the tissue. On a scale of 1-10, you'll be in the range of 8. Relax during your exercises.

When I began doing these exercises, I was barely able to endure the discomfort. If you continue to practice these exercises, you'll soon notice that your pain diminishes with each treatment.

You should be taking good care of your fascia every day. The return on investment for this investment is incomparable.

Exercise 1: SMR Lacrosse Chest Muscles

Begin by standing against the wall as shown in the image. The lacrosse ball should be placed against your body and then the wall. It is suggested to make use of a towel so that the ball can have greater grip against the wall.

Apply pressure on the ball until you are around eight on the scale of pain. Begin to gradually shift your body across the ball while maintaining the same amount of pressure.

Don't forget the pectoralis minor muscle that's situated in the top portion of your chest. It creates the shoulder joint.

Exercise 2 Foam Roll Lat

Your latissimus Dorsius muscle could be a factor in your pain. This workout is likely to feel like it was before!

In the end, you'll eventually be able to hold it when you roll for a couple of seconds. This is however an indication to start from here to the fullest extent.

Make sure you are in the lateral posture and put the foam roll into your armpit. Next, stretch your arm and then rotate your palms upwards. If you require more pressure, put your hand behind your head.

Lift your buttocks from the floor by shifting your weight to the feet that are placed. If you find this to be painful, you can start by placing the buttocks lying on the floor.

Begin to slowly move your body around the roll. Don't forget to breathe. If you require to take a break, relax for a few minutes and then resume the exercise.

Then, after two weeks, you'll be able to see that the workout became easy to perform.

Alternative:

Exercise 2: Lacrosse Lat Wall

If you find the exercise uncomfortable for you select a different method.

Lean forward against a wall. Your hands are in front of your head, and the ball is in your armpits. Be sure that the ball is against the wall, so that your tissue is easily reachable.

Now begin to move your upper body upwards and downwards on the ball.

Exercise 3: Lacrosse rotator cuff

This exercise is a must for the health of your shoulders!

It could take some time to find the best place to begin. If you find it, it may express its self by pulling in the shoulder's front and the arm. Typically, you can determine the exact location.

Set the ball down on a towel or mat so that it won't fall off during the workout.

Place yourself in a supine posture and place the ball below the back that is your arm. The area you're trying to find is just over the insertion into the muscle behind near the armpit.

You can try it. In most cases, you'll sense that you've found the perfect spot.

Then, you should set the arm in a 90 degree angle. If you'd prefer to push harder it is possible to turn your body toward the ball.

Then, move your shoulder forward and backwards by turning your arms towards your hips and your head.

Mobilization

By completing the exercises in the preceding chapters, you've built a foundation that is ideal for the care and repositioning of joints.

The aim of of the chapter in this section is to increase the range of motion of specific joints over time.

The flexibility of your shoulder joint is vital to maintaining the strength of your shoulders. Like other exercises, you'll only succeed if you practice these exercises daily.

The thoracic spine is mobile

In the earlier chapters, I've stressed that the importance of your thoracic spinal column for the health of your shoulder. A thoracic spinal structure that is flexible can form the foundation for the shoulder to be flexible. This is why the described method works for both of these areas.

Imagine that a movement restriction could have developed through time! It will take some time before you notice any improvement in the movement radius.

Training 1: Extension of the lacrosse pack

Make two lacrosse balls to prepare for this exercise. Attach them with adhesive tapes, such as duct tape, or packaging tape. Alternately, you could purchase a constructed construction like the one illustrated in the following photos.

The lacrosse pack should be placed on your back, so the spine of your between the two balls. The balls are positioned close to the spine on both sides.

The pack is situated in the lower region of your thoracic spine close to the first lumbar vertebra. Place your body in a supine position and rest your hands on your back. head.

Now, extend yourself as far as you can without lifting your buttocks off of the floor.

Once you've attained the maximum amount of movement you can do return to your beginning position and repeat the process twice more.

Then, you put the lacrosse bag just above the beginning point of two more locations along your spine.

Repeat the practice until the vertebrae in your thoracic spine are activated at least once.

This method is not the most pleasant, but it is very efficient in bringing some movement to your spine that is rusty.

2. Laying a rotation thoracic spine

In a lateral position, get into the posture and cross your leg to ensure that you can put it down on the floor.

In this workout, your head lies resting comfortably on a pillow, following the natural growth of your spine, if it is possible.

Then, grasp the inside of your knee of the leg that is crossed over by your hand, and raise it up to place it above your hips at an angle of 90 degrees. Place your leg on the floor throughout the exercise. Do this by placing your hand on your lower arm, rest it in the knee's hollow to avoid engaging your lumbar spine.

Then, wrap your ribs with your upper arm and then turn your body to the opposite side, without lifting your legs off of the ground. Every time you rotate you must exhale slowly and deeply.

Utilize the largest movement range throughout the rotation. Hold for approximately 1 second after the end Then go back to repeat.

Exercise 3 The Thoracic Spine Rotation and lateral flexion when sitting

This exercise is extremely efficient to increase the flexibility of your thoracic spine since it is a second plane of motion.

Lay down on the floor and then lay your legs on the floor so that your bottom feet are in line with each other.

If this is not possible you can simply rest your legs on top of your body while fully extended.

Then, you can cross your hands over your head. If it's more comfortable for you, simply place your hands upon your temples.

Then, rotate around the half-way mark of the movement margin. Bring your opposite elbow towards your knee. Reposition yourself and then move around the entire margin.

From here, move the elbow towards to the position of knee.

Alternate direction and repeat the process described in the two steps.

Shoulder mobilisation

We can now begin the stretching of the shoulders themselves. This particular exercise is not appropriate for every stage of the problem with the tendon. If the workout causes discomfort, take it off for the moment.

Exercise 4 Exercise 4: Snow angel

Place yourself in a supine posture then extend your arms towards the side at an angle of 90 degrees with your palms facing up.

Your elbow and arm should be pushed with a firm grip on the ground. Your shoulder blade should remain in touch with the floor throughout your entire workout!

Now, lift your arm upwards on the floor without your elbow or shoulder blade falling off with the floor.

Move your arm as high upwards as it is possible, and then hold your hands using the other hand to raise your head. Help lift your arm up even more.

Return to the beginning position and repeat.

Muscle Strengthening

The second part of the exercise program is dedicated to strengthening the muscles surrounding the shoulder joint.

While I'm usually an advocate of a rigorous training, it's best to not leave your ego in the cold as the performance of your body is what should be your primary goal with the exercises shown below!

By doing the exercises here that strengthen your muscles around the shoulder girdle won't only be strengthened, but the coordination or interplay between your muscles is enhanced through the stimulation.

The correct alignment of your muscles around your shoulder girdle are the most important factor to restore the proper shoulder mechanics.

These exercises are practiced using a ball that is a gymnastic or on any other surface with an elevated height.

I suggest first doing the exercise with no weights, however, you must be aware of an appropriate exercise performance. Later, you can use light dumbbells (1-3 kg).

1. Shoulder strength exercise exercise Y-T-

While your body is in a position, lie on the bench with your back facing downwards to ensure that your chest is at the top of your bench.

Now, raise your arms towards the front at an angle of 45 degrees and then to the side away the body. Your thumbs should be pointed upwards.

After the workout the shoulder blades should be close to one another and then be lowered.

Repeat this exercise prior to moving to another letter.

Then, you should bring your arms back with your elbow extended at 90 degrees. Your thumbs are always pointed upwards.

Your shoulder blades need to be as close as is possible, without compensating spinal vertebrae (your back is straight while you are on the benches).

Then, bend your elbows and then rotate your palms towards the front, so your thumbs point the back.

Move your bent arms towards the side of the position to ensure you shoulder blades are closer to one another.

Then bend your elbows until you reach 90 degrees, then the shoulder blades downwards and up.

From here, you simply move your shoulder around and then alternately move your back hand from forward to the rear.

Maintain the correct position of the shoulder blades.

Repeat the entire exercise before moving onto another letter.

Exercise 2 Exercise 2: Shoulder blade push-up

Make yourself into the push-up position. Let yourself sink the shoulder blades. ensure that your body is as steady as you can and keep your arms straight.

Your shoulder blades are at the bottom.

Now, pull yourself back into the original position using your arms extended.

If this workout is too difficult for you, start it by kneeling down on the floor.

Stretching

The static stretching routine usually consumes lots of time. So, I've limited my time in this chapter to exercises that have brought me and my clients the greatest benefits in the area in shoulder wellness.

This workout is extremely intense and particularly stretches the small pectoral muscle as well as your upper upper arm's front.

During the procedure it may cause the sensation of a tingling or numbness. sensation in the hands due to numerous nerves are able to pass through the area.

Exercise 1: Stretching your chest while lying down

Place yourself in a prone posture. Your arms are extended from you, in the shape of an Y.

Then, place your arms so that they are angled with your body. Repeat the process with your leg that is on the opposite side. Be sure to bend your leg in the event that you're unable to position your foot.

Turn the shoulder opposite to the arm stretched towards the floor.

Lift yourself up using the force of your leg and arm, then simultaneously you push your shoulder towards the ground.

If you experience shoulder pain, move your arm from the Y position to the T-position, and then test the exercise again.

Voodoo Floss

In the final portion in the course, we'll treat your tissue using the voodoo band once more. You'll notice the difference when you take off this band and putting it back on for the first time.

Voodoo's effects on the group are numerous and I've briefly mentioned them in the earlier chapter.

It is recommended that you have someone else to assist you in wrapping the band and also the performance in the practice. The band should be wrapped with an average tension of 50 75 - 75 percent.

I would suggest that you apply the appropriate tension carefully. The band must be removed following a 1-2 minutes.

A greater supply of blood is not advised and in extreme situations, could result in the destruction of tissues with a longer duration.

It is unlikely to be a problem for a healthy person within the context of an one-minute mobilization. I'll say it again to ensure that you are sure that nobody gets the notion that you have to put on the bracelet for more than 20 minutes. I suggest to take off the band immediately when you begin to get uncomfortable!

When you apply pressure to the skin, it will change to white, then return to the original color similar to sunburns.

If you rub your skin but the colour doesn't change back to the original color, it's the right time to take off the bandage.

1. Exercise: Voodoo shoulder floss

Begin in wrapping the band in the middle of your shoulder. Then, continue wrapping the band using half the width of the band and then overlapping to the shoulder. Then, stop when you have your upper arm totally covered by the band.

From there then wrap it up in an x-form . If there's any of the band remaining, secure it beneath an already-existing loop. Slowly, you can move your shoulder and arm completely or ask your companion to assist you in this.

Avoid areas where you experience shoulder discomfort. The force pushes into the tissue as the process progresses, and you can be uncomfortable.

Place your body down on the back, and place your arms at 90 degree angle in front of your body. Your partner holds your shoulder using his foot while you alternately turn your shoulder to the inside and outside.

As mentioned earlier, it could cause spots of red on your skin following the application of the bandage that will disappear within a few days.

Chapter 8: What Is The Cause Of Neck Pain?

There are many causes that can cause neck pain. A few of them include:

* Anomalies in joints or in bones - irregularities in bones or joints like dislocation of affected parts of our body may cause severe neck discomfort. These types of problems usually happen when someone is moving his head a lot and in a way that is not correct. The bones and joints of the neck area are less flexible than joints in other body parts. If the veins in the neck are a bit squeezed due to a lot of unintentionally moving, joints and bones could be affected, causing pain in the neck.

Poor posture - bad posture is among the most frequent causes of neck discomfort. The head weighs between 10 to 20 pounds. The muscles and tissues are complex and help to keep the head in position. When one stretches after a long period of poor posture muscles and tissues are likely to contract, causing discomfort in the neck.

* Stress and Trauma Additionally, there are emotional triggers that can lead to neck discomfort. Stress and trauma are only two of them. Like we said there are complex tissue and muscles that help keep your head in place. The muscles and tissues are linked to brain. Thus, whatever is being processed by the brain will travel through neck tissues and muscles before it gets to other organs of the body.

For instance, many of us know that stress levels could cause serious illness to our body. It could lead to serious ailments like heart failure. This is due to the pressure that the brain processes due to excessive thinking is flowing by the blood vessels. If you have a heart that is not strong it will break down before other organs will follow. However, before stress signals can reach the heart, they'll still need to travel through the neck muscles and tissues. Therefore, the next time you experience pain in your neck, perhaps it's an effect of trauma or tension.

* Tumors - Tumors can develop inside the neck. If neck pain persists for a long period

check to see whether there's a lump in your neck, which could require the attention of a specialist.

* Injuries , accidents as well as other injuries within the neck region can result in neck pain, but generally the pain will go disappears after a couple of hours, depending on the severity that the injury. However, certain neck pains caused by injuries , such as broken collar bones may be present for a few days or longer.

* Chronic or Acute Muscle Pain could also be the result from too much neck motion.

What is the cause of shoulder pain?

Similar to the neck, the shoulder is among the parts of your body that are constantly moving. Shoulder pains can be caused by:

* Strains caused by over exertion There are those who are a lot of work on the shoulders regular basis. Their bodies are accustomed to exerting themselves, so they do not feel so in discomfort. But if you're not moving as much, suddenly you began to work hard on your shoulders and arms you'll definitely be in pain.

* Tendonitis - it is a condition that occurs when the tendons become inflamed because of the stress of physical activity. There are various types of tendonitis that affect different areas in the human body. The type that causes shoulder discomfort is common for swimmers due to the fact that they are often using their shoulders.

* Instability of Joints and Shoulders The instability of the shoulders and joints is often due to weak bones, but it may also occur when joints are dislocated due to an injury or accident.

A fracture on Collar Bone - This can occur due to an accident.

* Frozen Shoulder is a condition like "stiff neck". It typically occurs after a night spent in a slouchy position. It will be like it is impossible to move your shoulders in a normal way the next day.

* Radiculopathy is a condition in which nerves are pinched because of an inefficient movement in the body.

How to prevent and get rid of neck pain

Tips to Avoid Neck Pain

* Rest in the right way Make sure to shut the windows before you fall asleep, particularly in the summer months. If temperatures drop in mid-night, chilling air causes your neck muscles to tighten and stiffen. Make sure to use the fan so you are able to sleep comfortably and rise the next day with stiff neck.

* Make sure to use the correct quantity of pillows. If you sleep with your back, do not add excessive pillows. If you're sleeping with your back on the ground, do not make use of too many pillows. If you are using excessive pillows for these sleeping positions your neck will be bent in a way that you experience a numb sensation as you wake up. The most comfortable position to sleep is to ensure that your head is in an even level.

Be careful when you are engaging in new activities. A number of people complain of neck pain after engaging in things they normally don't perform. They include gardening, focusing on at a new exercise or moving furniture, as well as packing items. Do a neck workout every day when you are doing heavy work that you would not normally perform. It is possible to follow the neck exercise below.

* Do Your Work Right If you are working at your the computer for long hours You must move your body regularly every several minutes. You should move your neck gently once at a time. Check out different directions for a short period of time. Alter your position from time to time. Make sure to stand and walk just a few feet away from your desk each 30 minutes. Try to work from a standing desk as much as you can.

Tips for Getting Rid of Neck Pain

Have you ever felt such neck pain that you thought you'd remove it? Neck pain can hinder you from working and doing the essential tasks of your day. There are many ways to alleviate neck discomfort. It is possible to do these yourself, even if your at home.

Therefore, if your neck pain isn't due to a serious injury, you can follow these steps to ease your neck discomfort in a matter of minutes.

* Neck Exercise Move your neck slowly between your arms. Make sure to do it with care so that you don't put pressure on your neck and cause additional discomfort. Then take your neck and move it gradually from one side to the other. Perform your back and forth movements after the side-to-side exercises in a row. Do not continue the exercise if you are experiencing discomfort when you move your neck.

* Shower Set the shower to hot. Your neck should be placed under the water that is lukewarm and let it run down your neck. Keep your neck submerged for five minutes. Keep your neck in a straight line when you are submerged.

* Make use of Bath Salts - bath salts have been proven to ease tensions in the muscles. Apply the bathing salts all over your neck in the

circular motion. Slowly rub the salts around your neck and notice the salts on your body.

* Heating Pad: place the heating pad around your neck and allow it to sit for around 15 to 30 minutes or as long as you feel the warmth. Heating pads can be helpful in stimulating blood flow , which makes you feel more relaxed after using one. Heating pads can be purchased at pharmacies.

* Ice Pack An ice pack can help to ease the neck pain. It is also possible to use bottles or a towel that you have placed in the freezer for about an hour.

* Request someone to rub Your Neck. Rubbing your neck often will help relax muscle and blood vessels.

Massage is the most relaxing and relaxing method of getting rid of neck discomfort. Each time you press your neck, it can help ease tension in your muscles and veins. You'll feel relaxed from stress after the massage.

* Meditate. Since neck pain can be result of stress, meditating can be an effective method

of relieving the discomfort. Relax your body. Try to imagine other things that aren't connected to your busy lifestyle toxic work and hectic schedule. Imagine beautiful things. Imagine a beautiful location. Spend at least 3 minutes in meditation, and you'll be more relaxed following that.

Life can be extremely difficult but you don't need to resent yourself for the mistakes that you cannot erase. Instead of contemplating the negatives, you can try something new that excites you. Have a night out with your others or take part in sporting activities. Do a run every morning or taking a swim lesson. These types of activities can aid in gaining fitness levels and distract your mind from your worries.

How to Avoid and eliminate Shoulder Pain

Tips to Avoid Shoulder Pain

Shoulder pain is a frequent problem for those who are constantly moving their shoulder during work. The pain might appear to be unnoticed during your working hours, but it can be felt at the end of your working hours and all you desire is to rest.

To prevent shoulder pain, here are a few useful suggestions to adhere to:

* Maintain a good posture - Keep an ideal posture, especially when sitting for long periods. You should move your shoulders each time after just a few minutes.

When going on long walks, do not wear high heels. If you are going to work wearing heels, put on flat shoes when traveling, and then put on your heels once you're working. When walking, make sure your shoulders do not pointing towards your ears. This practice is practiced by a lot of people, but they don't realize that it can strain the shoulder muscles, causing shoulder pain.

Read books If you are at home reading Try to keep a good posture while holding the book in a way that doesn't stress your shoulders. Be sure you're not leaning against the book when you read.

* When at work, do not sit for long periods of time. Take breaks every couple of minutes. Take a moment to stand and walk for a short distance and then return on your computer. Make sure to do this every day to ensure your blood circulation is maintained frequently.

Tips to Get Rid of Shoulder Pain

To ease shoulder pain, use these helpful tips:

* Shoulder exercise - grab an elastic band. Take each end and stretch it carefully. Keep the stretch position for around 30 seconds before releasing slowly. Repeat the exercise for 20 times. This is a form of resistance training program that will help strengthen and tone muscles on your shoulders. It can increase the flexibility and strength of your shoulders.

For the next workout you will need to fix the stretch band to something that resembles an incline. It should be approximately the same height as your waist. Keep your eyes away from the anchor, and then stretch the band by extending your arms to both sides. Keep your arms level. Don't let them hang over your ears. Keep them in the same position for a few seconds. After that, slowly lower your arms.

The final resistance exercise is back stretching. Make sure the stretching band is fixed to the stairway. Place the band in front of you and hold the ends by using both hands. Lengthen the band inwards. Slowly and be sure you don't allow your arms to reach above your shoulders. Keep your body in a straight line for at least five minutes. Lower the arms gradually. Repeat this exercise 15 times.

* Use a Hot Towel Soak the towel in warm water. Put the towel on your shoulders for a period of 20 minutes. After that, press your shoulders tightly using your thumb. Use the same pressure to the neck's bottom and your skull. If your shoulders are swollen then apply a cold compress after applying the hot compress. Allow it to remain for 20 minutes. Cold compresses will soothe the muscles and tissues that are swollen.

Regularly stretch your arms Do an arm-stretch workout each day. You can cross your fingers and raise your arms above your head until they're stretched. Keep them in this position for five second after which you can lower them. Perform a 20-second repetition of this.

* Cross Your Arms Cross one of your arms, then use your hand to pull the elbow of your extended arm toward your body. Keep this position for five second. Repeat the exercise 20 times.

* Shoulder Abduction Exercise - this workout requires you to lift a kilogram of weights. The weights are lifted over your head, and then hold it for 2 seconds. Repeat this 10 times. Then, lay on your stomach and lie on the floor on a firm and flat surface. Take the weights off of the ground and then raise them until they feel tension in your shoulders. Stay in the position for 2 seconds and repeat it ten times.

* Shoulder Rotation - lift your shoulders until your ears, and gradually lower them into your ribs. Repeat this exercise in the circular motion. Repeat for 20 times.

* Hot Bath - relax in a hot bath. The warm bath will relieve tension from your shoulders and help you relax.

* Massage Therapy: A massage therapist knows the best areas to apply pressure. He is aware of the amount of pressure your shoulder requires. Even if it is possible to massage your shoulders yourself but it's best to let someone else take care of it.

Herbal and Medical Treatments for shoulder and neck pain

The pain of shoulder and neck is not uncommon and happens to everyone. However, if you've been involved in an accident and your pain gets worse, medical treatment should be sought out. Talk to a doctor and explain your situation. The type of medication your doctor will prescribe will depend on the severity of your illness.

What should you do?

The first step you must do is prepare your mind and body. Remember that emotional issues could impact the physical body. If you're scared of having a physical exam, encourage yourself to believe you're the sole way to be well.

Here are a few medicines that your doctor might suggest to you. Knowing these points can aid you in preparing yourself prior to taking the treatment.

* Therapy - many doctors suggest this when your neck pain isn't due to any fractured bone. If the neck pain you are experiencing is due to nerve pinched or swelling and excessive movement, therapy is the most effective solution for you.

* Traction - This is an exercise that makes use of the pulleys as well as weights. The neck is stretched to stretch it out for a short period of immobilization. This treatment must be done with the guidance of the physical therapist or physician. This therapy is a fast treatment for neck discomfort.

* Temporary Immobilization for this type of treatment you'll need an elastic collar to take the neck from being strained. The collar is

used temporarily as a neck support for the head's weight. This is the most common treatment for those who have suffered an accident. It is recommended to use it for just a few days. A longer time of use could cause more damage to the neck.

* Acupuncture, a type of treatment, requires the use of needles. The needles are placed into various parts of the neck. Many kinds of pain can be relieved with the treatment of acupuncture. For the best results, you should test this type of treatment for a number of times.

* Steroid Injection - corticosteroid medication are injected close to the nerve root. The drugs will pass through your muscles and nerves to alleviate discomfort. Lidocaine, a numbing drug, can be used to alleviate neck discomfort. Antidepressants are also suggested by medical professionals.

* Surgery is the last thing your physician will recommend and only in cases of serious illness and requires a prompt solution. This only

applies to those who have suffered serious injuries like car crashes.

If your condition isn't severe, prescription drugs such as painkillers are sufficient to relieve the pain in your shoulder and neck. Herbal remedies can also be helpful in relieving shoulder and neck discomforts. People prefer natural solutions because they do not contain any chemical substances that are hidden. There is no need to be concerned about using them since you're aware that they don't cause any adverse effects.

* Sesame Seed Sesame Seeds - Black sesame seeds are the most effective. They have been proved to be effective in relieving any type of discomfort. You can take one handful of sesame seeds, and then soak them for a while in water. The sesame seeds should sit overnight. The next day, grab the spoonful of them and eat the seeds along with drinking a glass of water. It will be apparent that the pain will diminish within a couple of minutes.

Ghee is a butter that comes from South Asia. It is used to cook healthy meals. Ghee butter is used to treat ulcers and constipation. You can mix it into your meals or use as an alternative cooking oil. It helps to lubricate the joints that are dry inside your neck.

* Rhumatone Herbal Oil - this oil is a natural anti-inflammatory diet supplement that aids in the treatment of shoulder and neck discomforts. Rhumatone has formulated herbals which strengthen bones and allows muscles to move more comfortably. In addition to treating severe shoulder and neck pains, Rhumatone Herbal Oil is also beneficial in treating other health issues like neuralgia, arthritis and cervical spondylitis and other.

* Cloves from Garlic are an invigorating effect that assists in relaxing muscle and tendon. Garlic is cooked into hot mustard oil. Cook for about a minute. Put the garlic and oil in bottles. Let the oil mixture as well as garlic to settle. Rub the oil across your neck and shoulders. Massage gently and you will feel calm as the oil is taken in into your body.

* Essential Oil Essential oils are efficient in relaxing muscles that are strained. The best

remedy is chamomile oil. treatment for aching muscles. However lavender oil is most effective in releasing tension in joints and muscles. Marjoram oil can also be helpful for relieving muscles spasms. The other essential oils which can be effective in treating shoulder and neck problems are essential oils like tea tree, basil, and sage.

Honey and lemon juice Drinking lemon and honey juices can ease shoulder and neck discomfort. It is possible to utilize them as a replacement to cold and hot compresses as well as massage oils. Honey and lemon juices aid in the better digestion and elimination of toxin.

How To Handle The Pain

If you're in extreme pain, don't be afraid. The panic will only make you worse.

Here are a few efficient ways to manage the pain when in a position where immediate solution is not feasible:

Relax Your Mind - Try to concentrate. It is difficult when you're suffering, but it is important to attempt. Get rid of the negative thought patterns. Keep in mind that pain won't cause you to die. When your mind has calm, try the exercises described in the chapters Three and Four.

* Always be positive. Believing in the negative aspects of life only makes you feel more stressed. You already are aware that stress can trigger numerous health issues. Therefore, always be positive. If you've suffered an accident, remember that it's not an end in itself. Consider yourself fortunate that you're alive. Focus on building yourself from the loss you suffered.

* Always smile The act of smiling frequently will make you feel happier. Smile often and you'll feel more content than you actually are. So, if you continue to continue to smile even when you're feeling unwell then you'll eventually feel better.

* Laugh - a popular quote says that "Laughter is the most effective medicine." However, there's a doctor who says that this isn't true. According to him laughter is the most effective

remedy. Therefore, never stop laughing. But don't do it by yourself. Meet up with your buddies. Find people who will keep you laughing, particularly in times you're overwhelmed with issues.

These actions could not alleviate the problem immediately. However, living a life free of stress will avoid shoulder and neck discomforts from returning. In reality the shoulder and neck discomforts are only two of the physical issues you could be able to avoid if you lead in a healthy and happy life. Therefore, don't let anxiety, stress, heartbreak and stress to take over your life.

What should you be aware of about shoulder discomfort

Your shoulders are accountable for allowing your hands and arms with the entire range of motion they love. To be able to take advantage of the flexibility and flexibility that shoulders allow, they are prone to accidents and wear and wear and tear.

Know that the shoulders are among the joints with the greatest mobility within your body. This is why they are the most vulnerable. Some of the most common injuries that which can occur within the shoulder region are:

* Sprains

* Strains

* Dislocations

* Separations

* Tendinitis or Tendonitis? ?

* Bursitis

* Torn rotator cuffs

* Shoulders frozen

* Fragments

* Arthritis

If you are experiencing any issues however, it is always recommended to seek out a doctor to find the source of the issue, or at a minimum in order to determine if there is a problem that could be serious. Also, as when dealing with other health issues the shoulder problem is diagnosed using an established procedure:

* Discussing medical concerns and medical history with the doctor.

The doctor will then proceed to conduct a physical exam which tests your movement and restriction of movement you're experiencing in the affected region.

* Tests can be conducted by following methods:

Standard X-ray, specially used to diagnose fractures and other issues. Be aware it is important to note that soft tissues (like muscles) and tendons can't be detected by X-rays.

A medical history, in which patients inform the doctor about previous issues with the shoulder.

Ultrasound is the best non-invasive option, favored by many. A handheld scanner is placed against the skin to see the area affected.

O MRI (also known as Magnetic Resonance Imaging, or MRI is a different non-invasive technique that utilizes magnetic fields that are cross-sectional to produce an image view of your shoulder.

In this case, you should determine if you are suffering from any of the symptoms listed below or have experienced any of them in the past.-

* Shoulder pain especially during periods of relaxation.

* Shoulder pain that lasts more than a single day.

• It is difficult to raise your arms above your head.

It is possible to notice swelling and swelling on your arm.

* A weakness of the affected leg which makes the limb difficult for lifting heavy objects.

If you experience one of the symptoms listed above, they could be cause any of the following factors:--

* Inflammation of the muscles and tendons that surround the shoulder joint

* Torn, worn , or injured muscles or tendons.

* Separation of tendons and muscles from bone

* Stiffness in the shoulder

* Joint inflammation

* Calcium deposits

* Dislocation

* Injury

* Fracture

The typical shoulder pain sign and symptoms

Dislocation

They are one of the most prevalent problems with the shoulder that are faced by people who regularly exert a great deal of effort over their shoulders. Most often, they are caused by an intense external pull on the shoulder, causing the humerus's ball to break into the socket. The shoulder is pulled in a sudden manner and the surrounding muscles get taken off guard when it comes to protecting the socket in the shoulder. There are instances where shoulder dislocations occur frequently for some people. This is because of a condition known as shoulder instability.

* The signs and symptoms

Dislocations can happen in different directions: forward and backward, or downward or. Whatever the case the main issue is it is the shoulder that's in a bad its normal position, and it can cause extreme discomfort.

The symptoms will include:

Pain

Swelling

Muscle spasms

Numbing

Weakness

Bruising

* There are some situations when, after treatment, shoulders are more prone to

injuries. This is particularly the case for those who are younger and exposed to lots of sports and activities.

In the most extreme of cases it may require surgical intervention to fix worn or torn ligaments in order to prevent tearing and displacement of shoulder.

Separation

Separation happens when the collarbone, which forms a component of shoulder where it is in contact with the shoulder blade literally splits. The ligaments holding the joint together are torn in a way, either partially or all the way through, which causes the clavicle's position to shift. This is usually due to a powerful hit to the shoulder or a fall on a stretched hand.

www.ingramcontent.com/pod-product-compliance
Lightning Source LLC
Chambersburg PA
CBHW060223030426
42335CB00014B/1322